WHAT'S THE BEST MEDICINE FOR STAYING YOUNG? KNOWLEDGE.

DO YOU KNOW . . .

- THIN MEN WHO ARE OUT OF SHAPE ARE THREE TIMES MORE LIKELY TO DIE THAN OVERWEIGHT MEN *WHO EXERCISE*. SEE WHAT ELSE EXERCISE CAN DO TO KEEP YOU FIT AND FABULOUS.

- ALFALFA TEA IMPROVES BLOOD CIRCULATION TO THE BRAIN. THE RESULT? CLEARER THINKING, EVEN FOR ALZHEIMER'S SUFFERERS.

- TWO OUT OF THREE MEN HAVE INHERITED MALE-PATTERN BALDNESS. FORTUNATELY, A SIMPLE HAIR RINSE MADE WITH ARNICA OR SOUTHERNWOOD MAY HELP THEM HOLD ON TO THEIR HAIR.

- HALF THE PEOPLE OVER FIFTY SUFFER FROM . . . HEMORRHOIDS! DISCOVER HOW TO PREVENT THEM, AND HOW ACUPRESSURE CAN HELP RELIEVE THEM . . . FAST.

- MANY MEN KNOW THAT GINKGO AND GINSENG HELP COMBAT IMPOTENCE. BUT HAVE YOU HEARD OF YOHIMBINE? IT'S USED WIDELY IN PRESCRIPTION DRUGS, AND THE LOCAL HEALTH STORE HAS A NATURAL FORM OF IT TOO.

STOPPING TIME

Natural Remedies to Reverse Aging

Winifred Conkling

Foreword by
Kenneth Bernard Singleton, M.D., M.P.H.

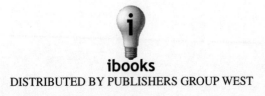

ibooks
DISTRIBUTED BY PUBLISHERS GROUP WEST

For Jonathan Rak,
the man I want
to grow old with

Contents

Foreword

One of the most exciting things that has happened in medicine in the past twenty years has been the explosion in research related to the aging process. As a result, we now have not only a much better understanding of how and why we age but a greater ability to intervene in that process (and actually reverse it in some cases).

Why the dramatic interest in aging in the past few years? One factor is that the baby boom generation—one of the most powerful economic forces in the nation—is getting older (and not liking the effects of aging on their bodies and health). As this generation ages, we physicians are seeing a growing number of patients complaining of symptoms associated with chronic degenerative diseases. In fact, our society is experiencing a literal epidemic of chronic degenerative diseases, such as adult-onset diabetes, arthritis, autoimmune disorders, cancer, heart disease, stroke, osteoporosis, and Alzheimer's disease.

Unfortunately, when it comes to treating the chronic complaints of aging, conventional medicine doesn't have a lot to offer. My training is in the specialty of internal medicine, and I can honestly tell you that for virtually all of the chronic degenerative diseases, when using mainstream medical treatments, my colleagues and I can do little more than "manage" our patients' symptoms and complaints. (Of course, we can occasionally effect a cure, but such cases are the exception, not the rule.) For most patients with degenerative diseases who seek help from Western physicians, the prognosis is for a slow progressive loss of function, despite the annual expenditure of billions of dollars in research for new and better treatments.

Since medical science seems ill equipped to handle the health consequences of aging, the questions become, What is causing the aging process, and How can we slow down or reverse it? Fortunately, much has been learned in recent years in answer to those questions. Based on these new findings, a new type of preventive medicine called "anti-aging medicine" has emerged. In addition to the techniques used by typical Western doctors, anti-aging medicine employs a number of natural methods of healing, including the use of herbal medicines, nutritional supplements, homeopathic remedies, and acupressure.

The goal of anti-aging medicine is not just to prolong life but also to delay—or avoid—the tremendous loss of function and well-being that comes with growing older. This aim was well stated a few years ago by a physician who said, "The goal of medicine should be to help people to grow old as late in life as possible." Why not at age 120?

Already much of his exciting research is being adopted by the American people. Consider the popularity of Dr. Dean Ornish's programs to reverse coronary heart disease and the booming sales of melatonin as an anti-aging therapy. According to *The New England Journal of Medicine,* approximately one-third of Americans seek out "alternative" practitioners in order to approach their health in a more holistic way.

Although traditional Western medicine has been slow to integrate these new anti-aging preventive principles into its patient care practices, things are changing. Every cardiologist I know is taking antioxidants (most commonly vitamin E). Other physicians are recommending that their patients use natural therapies for everything from Parkinson's disease to high cholesterol.

Things are changing, but don't wait for the doctors to lead the way. You are responsible for your health, and this book can help you take charge of it. The information presented here can help prevent and treat many common diseases and disorders associated with aging; in effect, it can help to slow down, stop, or even turn back the clock. This book is up-to-date in content and should be read by any serious person who truly desires to live longer—and live better.

Kenneth B. Singleton, M.D., M.P.H.
Internal Medicine
Preventive Medicine
Member, American Academy of Anti-Aging Medicine

Within every patient there resides a doctor and we as physicians are at our best when we put our patients in touch with the doctor inside themselves.

—Doctor and philosopher Albert Schweitzer
(1875–1965)

The healer of disease is Nature.

—Hippocrates

Introduction

We are all getting older, but some of us seem to be doing it more gracefully than others. You have probably met people who seem old at age 50, as well as those who seem young at age 85. While we all must adhere to the ticking of the same chronological clock, in large measure we have the freedom to set our own biological clock—the one that determines our functional age and dictates whether we look and act like we're 50 or 85.

You can stay young—and grow younger—by following a healthy lifestyle. You know the drill: Exercise regularly, eat a diverse and balanced diet, maintain a healthy weight, minimize stress. If you don't work at preserving your physical fitness, you will lose it. Beginning at age 40, the average person loses six pounds of muscle, 7 percent of heart function, and 8 percent of lung function every decade. This physical erosion is not inevitable. If you exercise regularly, you can build and maintain the muscle mass and strength of a 25-year-old, even if you're twice that age.

However, sooner or later time and genetics catch up with even the fittest among us. While physical conditioning can stave off many illnesses, as you get older you will experience some ailments and degenerative conditions. At those times, natural or "alternative" medicine can complement traditional health care, allowing you to take advantage of *all* the healing choices available to you.

How to Use This Book

Stopping Time is a comprehensive guide to natural treatments for a wide range of health problems common in people over age 40. By using a holistic approach to overall health, middle-aged and older people can lower their susceptibility to illness and live longer, healthier lives. The book is divided into three parts:

- Part I, "Growing Older, Naturally," offers an overview of the philosophy and practice of four major types of natural healing—herbal medicine, nutrition supplements, homeopathy, and acupressure.
- Part II, "Graying Gracefully," outlines specific lifestyle factors that can help improve your overall health, including exercise, diet, weight control, and relaxation techniques.
- Part III, "Natural Remedies A to Z," lists specific treatments for dozens of common illnesses and health problems. Each entry includes an overview of the illness, a thorough list of methods of natural healing, a section on prevention, and a list of warning signs. It also includes anecodotes and insights from professional healers, as well as resources for additional information.

The book can be read cover to cover or used as a reference when you're interested in learning about a specific medical condition. For example, if you're curious about the practice of homeopathy, you could turn directly to Chapter 4, "Homeopathy: The Dilution Solution," where you will find an overview of the history of homeopathy and an introduction to how it works. However, if you're interested in learning more about a specific medical condition, say osteoporosis, you could look it up in Part III. There you would find a description of the condition and the traditional ways it is treated, followed by specific prescriptive advice using natural medicine. The text also provides cross-references to background information and instructions in Parts I and II.

The information presented in this book is safe and accurate, but it does not replace the need for professional medical care. The suggestions listed here can help you work with your doctor to manage your health problems in a way that embraces the best of both conventional and alternative medical care.

PART ONE

GROWING OLDER, NATURALLY

CHAPTER 1

❧

Natural Medicine, Natural Cures: Following a Holistic Approach to Aging

Modern medicine can deliver miracles. A heart damaged by atherosclerosis can be rebuilt during bypass surgery; a pancreas that can no longer pump insulin can be supplanted by regular insulin injections; eyes clouded by cataracts can be surgically corrected with plastic lenses. While such man-made miracles offer great promise in many situations, there are other times when natural remedies can offer greater hope than conventional medicine can.

In recent years, a growing number of Americans have rediscovered the benefits of natural medicine. Disillusioned with the often ineffective invasiveness of many conventional treatments, many open-minded people have turned to practitioners of natural medicine for help. Allopathic medicine—the term used to refer to conventional Western medicine—is superb at dealing with trauma and bacterial infections, but it is not nearly as effective with chronic pain, autoimmune disease, and degenerative conditions. These limitations have led to a greater acceptance of alternative approaches to healing. In fact, a 1993 study published in *The New England Journal of Medicine* reported that an astounding one out of every three respondents to a survey had consulted at least one herbalist, homeopath, dietary counselor, or other practitioner of natural medicine in 1990.

Natural medicine is based on the simple—but profound—belief that the human body has an amazing ability to heal itself. The practitioner's role is to assist the body in the healing process, not simply to suppress the symptoms of disease. As part of this philosophy, the body must be viewed holistically: The practitioner must focus on the overall condition of the patient, not just the part that is injured or sick. By contrast, conventional physicians tend to deal with the symptoms of a disease rather than its root cause.

You don't have to choose between conventional medicine and natural medicine; instead, you can borrow the best of both approaches to healing and customize them to your particular situation. Of course, let your conventional physician and your practitioner of natural medicine know about each other. In some cases, the treatments provided by one may conflict with those of the other; for example, an herbal remedy might undermine the effectiveness of a prescribed drug or vice versa. In the end, a cooperative approach that includes both traditional treatments and natural remedies will probably provide the best care for your overall health.

Medical Musts: Screening Tests, Exams, and Immunizations

While natural remedies can be helpful in the treatment and management of disease, you must know you have a health problem before you can treat it. In most cases, these diagnostic tests should be performed by a conventional physician.

It's heartbreaking to receive a diagnosis of a serious illness, but it is particularly difficult when the problem could have been controlled or reversed if only it had been caught at an earlier stage. The best way to detect a medical problem in its early, treatable stages is to have regular medical exams and screening tests, as well as vaccinations. While sometimes unpleasant, these tests, exams, and vaccinations really can save your life. Some 50,000 to 70,000 people die of influenza, pneumonia, or hepatitis B in the United States every year, and about half of those deaths could be prevented by vaccination. The older you are, the more important it is to keep your vaccinations up-to-date, since immunity declines with age.

Screening Tests and Exams

These tests should be routinely performed; others may be necessary if recommended by your physician or if your medical history dictates:

- **Blood pressure measurement:** Annually after age 50; more often if under treatment for hypertension. (Blood pressure is taken as part of a routine physical exam. Between physicals, you may want to test your blood pressure yourself; many pharmacies and grocery stores have machines available for public use.)
- **Breast exam** (women): Monthly at home; annually by your doctor.
- **Cholesterol:** Every five years after age 50; more often if you have a history of atherosclerosis or coronary disease, or if your total cholesterol levels exceed 200 milligrams per deciliter (for men) or 240 milligrams per deciliter (for women).
- **Complete physical:** Every five years up to age 60; every two years to age 65; annually thereafter.
- **Dental exam and tooth cleaning:** Every six months; more often if periodontal disease is present.
- **Dental X rays:** Every two to three years.
- **Electrocardiogram:** Every three years after age 50; more often if there is evidence of heart disease.
- **Eye examination:** Every two years.
- **Mammogram** (women): Every one to two years between ages 40 and

49; annually age 50 and older. If you have a family history of breast cancer, a mammogram may be recommended even earlier.

- **Occult blood in stool:** Annually after age 50.
- **Pelvic exam** (women): Annually, including a Pap smear.
- **Prostate exam** (men): Annually. The prostate-specific antigen (PSA) test can detect prostate cancer early, though it's not always clear what to do with the information. Some physicians reserve the PSA test for those men with a strong family history of the disease. Many recommend an annual PSA test (along with a digital rectal exam) beginning at age 50– or 40, if the patient is at high risk.
- **Rectal exam/digital:** Annually after age 40.
- **Sigmoidoscopy:** Every three to five years after age 50.
- **Skin exam:** Once a month, using a mirror or asking a friend for help, check every square inch of your skin for abnormalities, including moles, rashes, or scaling. Annually, have a dermatologist perform a skin check, starting at age 40, or earlier if you have a lot of sun-related skin damage.
- **Testicular exam** (men): Annually.

Immunizations

ANNUAL
- **Influenza:** Flu shots are recommended for all people over age 65; nursing home residents; and younger people who have diabetes, heart or lung disease, kidney or liver disease, immune system disease, or any other chronic medical condition. *Note:* The vaccine should be avoided by people who are allergic to eggs, because the virus is grown in eggs. Talk to your doctor about alternative immunization.

EVERY TEN YEARS
- **Tetanus and diphtheria:** This vaccine is recommended for all adults who have not been immunized or who are due for a booster. Initially, the combined vaccine should be given in three doses, the second one four weeks after the first, and the third one six to twelve months after the second. After that, a booster should be given every ten years. A tetanus booster also should be given whenever a person has a large, deep cut or puncture wound that could have been contaminated by dirt. By age 60, fewer than half of Americans have protective levels of tetanus antibodies. Since older people account for the majority of tetanus cases, it's especially important for them not to fall behind on boosters.

ONE TIME ONLY

- **Pneumococcal pneumonia:** This vaccine is recommended for all people over age 65, as well as alcoholics and younger adults with diabetes, heart or lung disease, or other chronic illness that could make them more susceptible to complications of pneumonia. Also people aged 50 and over in group-living facilities.

- **Rubella (German measles):** This vaccine is recommended for all adults who do not know whether they received the live-virus vaccine, as well as those whose blood tests fail to show immunity to the disease. *Note:* This immunization is not recommended for people with an immune system disorder.

- **Hepatitis B:** This vaccine is recommended for all adults at risk of exposure to hepatitis B, including health care workers, hemophiliacs, and people who receive blood transfusions or blood products, family members of people with the disease, and male homosexuals.

Finding a Practitioner

Naturopathic physicians practice natural medicine, using a variety of healing techniques, including herbalism, homeopathy, nutrition supplementation, and acupressure. (Some practitioners specialize in just one field; for information on herbalists, see page 14; on nutritionists, page 34; on homeopaths, page 58; and acupressurists and acupuncturists, page 75.)

Training to become a naturopath resembles traditional medical training. Standard premed courses must be taken by students at the nation's three recognized naturopathic medical schools, Bastyr University, the National College of Naturopathic Medicine, and the Southwest College of Naturopathic Medicine and Health Sciences. Students take many of the same courses as conventional medical students, as well as courses in clinical nutrition, herbal medicine, physical medicine, and counseling.

For a referral to a naturopath or a medical doctor who specializes in natural treatments, contact:

American Association of Naturopathic Physicians
2366 Eastlake Avenue E. Suite 322
Seattle, WA 98102

National College of Naturopathic Medicine
11231 S.E. Market Street
Portland, OR 97216
(503) 255-4860

CHAPTER 2

❧

Healing Herbs:
Harvesting Mother Nature's Medicines

Mother Nature offers almost everything you need to stock
your medicine cabinet. Herbal remedies (or botanicals)
can be used to treat most common conditions and ailments. They are often safer, cheaper, and more effective
than synthetic drugs, and they can be used to treat a hand-
ful of conditions that mainstream medicines can't touch,
such as viral infections like influenza. That's not to say that
man-made drugs have no place in your medicine cabinet;
they do. But in many cases herbal remedies can complement conventional medicine and add another dimension to
your health care.

Every culture on Earth has relied on the natural healing
ability of plants to treat almost every ailment, from conditions associated with infancy to those of old age. World-
wide, four out of five people use herbs as the basis of their
medical care. Though most Americans rely on synthetic
drugs produced in a laboratory, European doctors often

prescribe herbal treatments for their patients. In fact, half of the prescriptions German doctors write for depression are for St. John's wort, an herb, rather than for man-made psychoactive drugs.

One of the main reasons that synthetic medicines are more popular than herbs in the United States is that drug companies can patent those drugs they create, but they cannot patent Mother Nature's cures. Still, about 25 percent of all prescription drugs sold in the United States contain active ingredients isolated from plants, and most synthetic drugs are little more than laboratory versions of chemicals that occur naturally in plants. Consider pseudoephedrine, the active ingredient in many cold and allergy medications. This chemical is actually a synthetic version of ephedrine, a natural decongestant found in the herb ephedra. Painkillers such as morphine or codeine are derived from the opium poppy; the cancer drugs vincristine and vinblastine come from periwinkle; and even old-fashioned aspirin finds its origins in the salicin in willow bark.

Many drug companies believe that the so-called "wonder drugs" of the future may have their roots in botanical medicines. In fact, the pharmaceutical giant Pfizer is currently working with the China Academy of Traditional Chinese Medicine in Beijing to collect and study the active ingredients in the herbs used in traditional Chinese medicine. The company is also working with the New York Botanical Garden in the Bronx to study the disease-fighting properties of various plants found in the United States.

Strong Medicine

Many people who agonize over taking an over-the-counter painkiller think nothing of swallowing an herbal treatment because they consider it "natural" and therefore not dangerous. But herbs that have the ability to heal also have the ability to harm, if misused. Yes, in general herbal remedies are safer and have fewer side effects than man-made drugs, but they can be as potent and harmful as synthetic drugs, and they should be treated with the same respect. Like any other drugs, herbs can have negative and sometimes dangerous side effects if taken in excessive doses. Consider coffee, America's favorite beverage and most widely used herb. (Yes, coffee is a botanical.) For most people, drinking one or two cups of coffee a day won't cause any problems, but four or five cups can cause headaches and nervousness, and ten or fifteen cups can cause dizziness, ringing in the ears, or even temporary hearing loss. When it comes to herbs—as with many things—more is not necessarily better.

Part of the confusion about safety stems from the way herbal treatments are labeled. Unlike synthetic drugs, herbal remedies do not have to go through the formal approval process of the U.S. Food and Drug Administration because they are classified as foods or food additives rather than drugs. This means that manufacturers of herbal remedies must be cautious about the claims they make on package labels—drug-related claims and warnings are prohibited. Consumers must be on their toes about understanding the products they are buying. It's up to you to read the package directions; always follow the dosage information on the product label. If you have any questions about how a product should be used, contact the manufacturer for more information.

You can find many herbal remedies in health food stores, but recently they have been showing up in conventional supermarkets and pharmacies as well. If you can't find what you need at local stores, refer to page 15 for information on mail-order companies that sell herbs.

Most of the herbal treatments listed in this book involve single herbs rather than formulas, or blends of herbs designed to act synergistically to achieve specific results for a specific individual. Some herbal formulas can be found at health food stores; others must be prepared by a professional herbalist.

Using Herbs

While all herbal medicines use plant material, different medicines employ different parts of the plant, such as the leaves, seeds, flowers, roots, bark, or berries. The various "recipes" have been refined and improved by herbalists over thousands of years. Though only a tiny fraction of the world's plants have been tested for their medicinal potential, American herbalists use approximately one thousand different herbs to treat everything from Alzheimer's disease to varicose veins.

Regardless of what plants they are made of, herbal medicines come in one of several forms, including:

- Teas: Made by steeping about 1 teaspoon of dried herbs or 3 teaspoons of fresh herbs in 1 cup of boiling water for 5 minutes or so, then straining. Most herbal teas are not strong enough to have medicinal value.
- Infusions: Made much the same way as strong tea, with several important exceptions. The water should be just short of boiling (since boiling water disperses important volatile oils in the steam), and the herbs are steeped for 20 to 30 minutes, so the resulting liquid is much more potent and often more bitter. The infusion should be strained before drinking. Most infusions are made with ½ to 1 rounded teaspoon of dried herb or 3 teaspoons of fresh herb per cup of water. The standard dose is ½ cup, three times a day.
- Decoctions: Made like infusions, only the bark, roots, or berries of the herbs are simmered (never boiled), rather than merely steeped, for 20 to 30 minutes (or sometimes longer). Most decoctions are made with ½ to 1 rounded teaspoon of dried herb per cup of water. The standard dose is ½ cup, three times a day.
- Tinctures: Made by soaking herbs in an alcohol solution (25 percent alcohol/75 percent water) for a specified period of time (from several hours to several days, depending on the herb). Commercial tinctures

use ethyl alcohol, but apple cider vinegar, vodka, brandy, and rum are suitable for home use (and the brandy and rum can help to disguise the bitter favor of some herbs). Because alcohol acts as a preservative, tinctures can be stored for up to two years. Use 1 ounce of crushed dried herbs with 5 ounces of distilled spirits. When preparing a tincture, shake the mixture every few days to encourage alcohol uptake of the herb's active ingredients. *Warning:* Do not use methyl alcohol or isopropyl alcohol (rubbing alcohol) when making tinctures; they are toxic if taken internally.

- Extracts: Made by distilling some of the alcohol from a tincture, leaving a more potent concentrate behind. Most commercial extracts use vacuum distillation or filtration techniques, which do not require the use of high temperatures.
- Powder: Made by removing the moisture from an extract, then grinding the solid herbal concentrate into granules or powders, which can be shaped into capsules or tablets.

Most of the herbal treatments mentioned in this book involve infusions or decoctions, which may have a sharp, bitter taste. If you don't care for the flavor of an herbal remedy, try masking it with sugar, honey, lemon, fruit juice, or even flavored tea mix. You can also purchase prepared tinctures, extracts, or powdered herbs and follow the dosage information on the product labels.

Before using herbs, check with your doctor, since herbal medicines can interact with conventional drugs. Use only the recommended amounts, and take herbs only for the recommended time periods. The risk of side effects goes up when people take large amounts of herbs for extended periods. Start with a low-strength preparation and strengthen it only if necessary.

Watch out for symptoms of overdose or toxicity. Typical symptoms include stomach upset, nausea, diarrhea, or headache an hour or two after taking an herb. If you develop any suspicious symptoms after taking an herb, stop taking it and see if the symptoms disappear. If you have an adverse reaction, report it to the FDA's MedWatch office at (800) 332-1088.

Finding a Qualified Herbalist

The states do not certify or license herbalists, so it's up to you to check the credentials of any practitioner you consult. Look for someone who is a member of the American Herbalists Guild, or if you're considering a naturopathic physician or acupuncturist who uses herbs, make sure that person meets the necessary requirements for licensing in your state.

For more information on herbal medicine and referrals to practitioners in your area, contact:

American Herbalists Guild
P.O. Box 1683
Soquel, CA 95073
(408) 464-2441
(408) 469-4372

American Association of Naturopathic Physicians
2366 Eastlake Avenue E., Suite 322
Seattle, WA 98102
(206) 323-7610

Additional publications, newsletters, and books on herbal medicine are available from:

American Foundation of Traditional Chinese Medicine
505 Beach Street
San Francisco, CA 94133
(415) 776-0502

American Botanical Council
P.O. Box 201660
Austin, TX 78720
(512) 331-8868
(800) 373-7105

Herb Research Foundation
1007 Pearl Street, Suite 200
Boulder, CO 80302
(303) 449-2265

Institute for Traditional Medicine
2017 Southeast Hawthorne
Portland, OR 97214
(503) 233-4907

Herb manufacturers with mail-order catalogs include:

Earth's Harvest
2557 N.W. Division
Gresham, OR 97030
(800) 428-3308

East Earth Trade Winds
P.O. Box 493151
Redding, CA 96049-3151
(800) 258-6878
(916) 241-6878 in California

Eclectic Institute
14385 Lusted Rd.
Sandy, OR 97055
(800) 332-HERB

Herb-Pharm
P.O. Box 116
William, OR 97544
(503) 846-6262

Herbs of Grace
Division of School of Natural Medicine
P.O. Box 7369
Boulder, CO 80306-7369
(303) 443-4882

Meridian Traditional Herbal Products
44 Linden Street
Brookline, MA 02146
(800) 356-6003
(617) 739-2636 in Massachusetts

McZand Herbal
P.O. Box 5312
Santa Monica, CA 90409
(310) 822-0500

Nature's Way Products
10 Mountain Springs Parkway
Springville, UT 84663
(801) 489-1520

Windriver Herbs
P.O. Box 3876
Jackson, WY 83001
(800) 903-HERB

Herbs Used to Treat Common Ailments

Thousands of herbs are used for healing, but most Western herbalists regularly use fewer than 200 in their prescriptions. The following list includes a number of herbs used to treat the ailments discussed in this book. This herb list is cross-referenced with the ailments listed in Part III. You may be surprised to learn that one herb can be used in the treatment of a number of unrelated conditions. Possible side effects are noted, but they are extremely uncommon at the doses recommended in this book. Pregnant women should not use any herbs without contacting a physician, but those herbs most likely to cause problems during pregnancy are noted.

ALFALFA *(Medicago sativa)*
USED TO TREAT: Alzheimer's disease (page 139), cancer (page 186), osteoarthritis (page 165), rheumatoid arthritis (page 175)
SIDE EFFECTS: Diarrhea, nausea
PRECAUTION: Do not eat alfalfa seeds, which contain a toxic amino acid that can cause blood-clotting problems

ALOE VERA *(Aloe vera)*
USED TO TREAT: Constipation (page 221), periodontal disease (page 371)
SIDE EFFECTS: None when used externally; intestinal cramps, diarrhea when used internally
PRECAUTION: Generally a safe herb

ANGELICA *(A. atropurphurea)*
USED TO TREAT: Anemia (page 148), osteoarthritis (page 165), rheumatoid arthritis (page 175)
SIDE EFFECTS: Skin rash
PRECAUTION: Generally a safe herb

ANISE *(Pimpinella anisum)*
USED TO TREAT: Prostate cancer (page 186)
SIDE EFFECTS: Migraine headache, abnormal blood clotting
PRECAUTION: Women should avoid during pregnancy

APPLE *(Malus sylvestris)*
USED TO TREAT: Colon cancer (page 186)
SIDE EFFECTS: Diarrhea; avoid eating the seeds, which contain the poison cyanide
PRECAUTION: Generally a safe herb

ARNICA *(Arnica montana)*
USED TO TREAT: Hair loss (page 268)
SIDE EFFECTS: Skin irritation
PRECAUTION: Generally a safe herb

BARBERRY *(Berberis vulgaris)*
USED TO TREAT: Gallbladder disease (page 256), hypertension (page 304), osteoarthritis (page 165), rheumatoid arthritis (page 175)
SIDE EFFECTS: Convulsions, nausea, uterine contractions, vomiting
PRECAUTION: Avoid during pregnancy

BASIL *(Ocimum basilicum)*
USED TO TREAT: Depression (page 236), hysterectomy recovery (page 313)
SIDE EFFECTS: Nausea, vomiting, uterine contractions
PRECAUTION: Avoid during pregnancy

BILBERRY *(Vaccinium myrtillus)*
USED TO TREAT: Cataracts (page 205)
SIDE EFFECTS: Lowers blood sugar levels
PRECAUTION: Diabetics should not use this herb without professional supervision

BLACK COHOSH *(Cimicifuga racemosa)*
USED TO TREAT: Prostate cancer (page 186), meno-

pausal symptoms (page 340), osteoarthritis (page 165), rheumatoid arthritis (page 175)
SIDE EFFECTS: Diarrhea, dizziness, headache, joint pain, nausea, slow heart rate, vomiting
PRECAUTION: Pregnant women and people with heart disease should avoid this herb

BLACK HAW *(Viburnum prunifolium)*
USED TO TREAT: Osteoarthritis (page 165), rheumatoid arthritis (page 175)
SIDE EFFECTS: Nausea, tinnitus, vomiting
PRECAUTION: Avoid during pregnancy

BLACKBERRY *(Rubus fruticosus)*
USED TO TREAT: Hemorrhoids (page 299)
SIDE EFFECTS: Nausea, vomiting
PRECAUTION: Generally a safe herb

BONESET *(Eupatorium perfoliatum)*
USED TO TREAT: Flu (page 213)
SIDE EFFECTS: Diarrhea, nausea, vomiting
PRECAUTION: In large amounts this herb can cause liver damage

BOSWELLIA *(Boswellia serrata)*
USED TO TREAT: Osteoarthritis (page 165), rheumatoid arthritis (page 175)
SIDE EFFECTS: None known
PRECAUTION: Generally a safe herb

BUTCHER'S BROOM *(Ruscus aculeatus)*
USED TO TREAT: Varicose veins (page 392)
SIDE EFFECTS: None known
PRECAUTION: Generally a safe herb

CALIFORNIA POPPY *(Eschscholzia californica)*
USED TO TREAT: Insomnia (page 332)
SIDE EFFECTS: None known
PRECAUTION: Generally a safe herb

Cascara sagrada *(Rhamnus purshiana)*
USED TO TREAT: Constipation (page 221)
SIDE EFFECTS: Intestinal cramping
PRECAUTION: This herb should not be used for more than two weeks; over time it can cause "lazy bowel" syndrome

Celery *(Apium graveolens)*
USED TO TREAT: Hypertension (page 304)
SIDE EFFECTS: Potassium deficiency
PRECAUTION: Avoid during pregnancy

Chamomile *(Matricaria chamomilla)*
USED TO TREAT: Bronchitis (page 213), colds (page 213)
SIDE EFFECTS: Nausea, vomiting
PRECAUTION: People allergic to ragweed should avoid this herb

Club moss *(Huperzia serrata)*
USED TO TREAT: Alzheimer's disease (page 139)
SIDE EFFECTS: None known
PRECAUTION: Generally a safe herb

Coffee *(Coffea arabica)*
USED TO TREAT: Obesity (page 352)
SIDE EFFECTS: Anxiety, elevated heart rate, high blood pressure, insomnia
PRECAUTION: Generally a safe herb

Comfrey *(Symphytum officinale)*
USED TO TREAT: Osteoporosis (page 358)
SIDE EFFECTS: Stomach upset
PRECAUTION: This herb can cause liver damage at high doses

Cypress *(Cupressus sempervirens)*
USED TO TREAT: Incontinence (page 324)
SIDE EFFECTS: None known
PRECAUTION: Generally a safe herb

DANDELION *(Taraxacum officinale)*
USED TO TREAT: Cancer (page 186), gallbladder disease (page 256), heart disease (page 283), menopausal symptoms (page 340), obesity (page 352)
SIDE EFFECTS: Skin rash
PRECAUTION: Generally a safe herb

DEVIL'S CLAW *(Harpagophytum porcumbens)*
USED TO TREAT: Gout (page 262), osteoarthritis (page 165), rheumatoid arthritis (page 175)
SIDE EFFECTS: None known
PRECAUTION: Generally a safe herb

ECHINACEA *(Echinacea angustifolia)*
USED TO TREAT: Bronchitis (page 213), cancer (page 186), colds (page 213), flu (page 213), toothache (page 228)
SIDE EFFECTS: Tingling on tongue
PRECAUTION: Generally a safe herb

EPHEDRA *(Ephedra sinica)*
USED TO TREAT: Obesity (page 352)
SIDE EFFECTS: Dry mouth, heart palpitations, high blood pressure, insomnia
PRECAUTION: People with high blood pressure should avoid this herb

EUCALYPTUS *(Eucalyptus globulus)*
USED TO TREAT: Burning feet (page 250)
SIDE EFFECTS: Skin rash
PRECAUTION: Do not take internally

FENUGREEK *(Trigonella foenum-graecum)*
USED TO TREAT: Diabetes (page 243), menopausal symptoms (page 340), osteoarthritis (page 165), rheumatoid arthritis (page 175)
SIDE EFFECTS: Nausea, uterine contractions, vomiting
PRECAUTION: Avoid during pregnancy

FRINGE TREE *(Chionanthus virginicus)*
USED TO TREAT: Gallbladder disease (page 256)
SIDE EFFECTS: None known
PRECAUTION: Generally a safe herb

GARLIC *(Allium sativum)*
USED TO TREAT: Alzheimer's disease (page 139), anxiety (page 159), bronchitis (page 213), cancer of the stomach (page 186), colds (page 213), diabetes (page 243), flu (page 213), heart disease (page 283), hypertension (page 304)
SIDE EFFECTS: Clotting disorders, skin rash
PRECAUTION: Generally a safe herb

GINKGO *(Ginkgo biloba)*
USED TO TREAT: Alzheimer's disease (page 139), cancer (page 186), hearing loss (page 274), heart disease (page 283), impotence (page 318)
SIDE EFFECTS: Clotting disorders, diarrhea, restlessness
PRECAUTION: Generally a safe herb

GINSENG *(Panax quinquefolius)*
USED TO TREAT: Cancer (page 186), diabetes (page 243), impotence (page 318)
SIDE EFFECTS: Breast soreness, elevated blood pressure, insomnia
PRECAUTION: Generally a safe herb

GOLDENSEAL *(Hydrastis canadensis)*
USED TO TREAT: Periodontal disease (page 371), toothache (page 228)
SIDE EFFECTS: High blood pressure, skin irritation
PRECAUTION: People with high blood pressure should avoid this herb

GOTU KOLA *(Centella asiatica)*
USED TO TREAT: Varicose veins (page 392)
SIDE EFFECTS: Skin rash
PRECAUTION: Generally a safe herb

HAWTHORN *(Crataegus oxyacantha)*
USED TO TREAT: Angina (page 154), heart disease (page 283), hypertension (page 304)
SIDE EFFECTS: Low blood pressure, sedation
PRECAUTION: Avoid during pregnancy

HOPS *(Humulus lupulus)*
USED TO TREAT: Insomnia (page 332)
SIDE EFFECTS: Skin rash
PRECAUTION: Generally a safe herb

HOREHOUND *(Marrubium vulgare)*
USED TO TREAT: Pneumonia (page 377)
SIDE EFFECTS: Diarrhea, nausea
PRECAUTION: People with heart disease should avoid this herb because in high doses it can cause cardiac arrhythmias

HORSE CHESTNUT *(Aesculus hippocastanum)*
USED TO TREAT: Varicose veins (page 392)
SIDE EFFECTS: Skin irritation
PRECAUTION: Seed coating can be toxic if not removed

HORSETAIL *(Equisetum arvense)*
USED TO TREAT: Osteoporosis (page 358)
SIDE EFFECTS: Fever, muscle weakness
PRECAUTION: Avoid during pregnancy

HUANG QI *(Astragalus membranaceus)*
USED TO TREAT: Incontinence (page 324)
SIDE EFFECTS: None known
PRECAUTION: Generally a safe herb

HYSSOP *(Hyssopus officinalis)*
USED TO TREAT: Pneumonia (page 377)
SIDE EFFECTS: None known
PRECAUTION: While this herb has not been shown to stimulate uterine contractions, it has been used in some cultures to induce abortion; avoid during pregnancy

JUNIPER *(Juniperus communis)*
USED TO TREAT: Osteoarthritis (page 165), rheumatoid arthritis (page 175)
SIDE EFFECTS: Blood in urine, diarrhea, high blood pressure, kidney irritation
PRECAUTION: People with kidney problems or a kidney infection should avoid this herb

KING'S CLOVER *(Melilotus officinalis)*
USED TO TREAT: Varicose veins (page 392)
SIDE EFFECTS: Clotting problems
PRECAUTION: Do not use in combination with blood-thinning drugs

LICORICE *(Glycyrrhiza glabra)*
USED TO TREAT: Bronchitis (page 213), cancer (page 186), colds (page 213), menopausal symptoms (page 340)
SIDE EFFECTS: High blood pressure, hormone imbalances, muscle weakness
PRECAUTION: People with high blood pressure should avoid this herb

MARJORAM *(Origanum majorana)*
USED TO TREAT: Toothache (page 228)
SIDE EFFECTS: None known
PRECAUTION: Generally a safe herb

MEADOWSWEET *(Filipendula ulmaria)*
USED TO TREAT: Osteoarthritis (page 165), rheumatoid arthritis (page 175)
SIDE EFFECTS: Stomach upset, tinnitus, uterine contractions
PRECAUTION: Avoid during pregnancy

MISTLETOE *(Phoradendron serotinum)*
USED TO TREAT: Cancer (page 186)
SIDE EFFECTS: Coma, convulsions, slow heart rate

PRECAUTION: Do not use berries, which are toxic; avoid during pregnancy

MOTHERWORT *(Leonurus cardiaca)*
USED TO TREAT: Heart disease (page 283)
SIDE EFFECTS: Clotting disorders, skin rash
PRECAUTION: People with clotting disorders and pregnant women should avoid this herb

NETTLE *(Urtica dioica)*
USED TO TREAT: Gout (page 262)
SIDE EFFECTS: Stomach upset, urinary retention
PRECAUTION: Women should avoid during pregnancy

OATS *(Avena sativa)*
USED TO TREAT: Depression (page 236)
WARNING: Do not use if sensitive to gluten
PRECAUTION: Generally a safe herb

PARSLEY *(Petroselinum crispum)*
USED TO TREAT: Bad breath (page 182)
SIDE EFFECTS: Skin rash
PRECAUTION: Generally a safe herb

PASSIONFLOWER *(Passiflora incarnata)*
USED TO TREAT: Insomnia (page 332)
SIDE EFFECTS: Uterine contractions
PRECAUTION: Avoid during pregnancy

PEPPERMINT *(Mentha spp.)*
USED TO TREAT: Facial wrinkles (page 398)
SIDE EFFECTS: Skin irritation
PRECAUTION: Peppermint can decrease milk flow in nursing mothers

PILEWORT *(Ranunculus ficaria)*
USED TO TREAT: Hemorrhoids (page 299)
SIDE EFFECTS: Skin irritation
PRECAUTION: Do not take internally

Primrose oil *(Primula spp.)*
USED TO TREAT: Hot flashes (page 340)
SIDE EFFECTS: Stomach upset
PRECAUTION: Pregnant women, people on blood-thinning drugs, and those allergic to aspirin should avoid this herb

Psyllium *(Plantago psyllium)*
USED TO TREAT: Constipation (page 221)
SIDE EFFECTS: Diarrhea, stomach upset
PRECAUTION: Generally a safe herb

Red clover *(Trifolium pratense)*
USED TO TREAT: Cancer (page 186)
SIDE EFFECTS: Blood clots
PRECAUTION: This herb should be avoided by women taking birth-control pills and people with heart disease or a history of stroke

Red pepper *(Capsicum annuum)*
USED TO TREAT: Burning feet (page 250); broken, cracked, or chipped teeth (page 228)
SIDE EFFECTS: Skin rash
PRECAUTION: Generally a safe herb

Rhubarb *(Rheum officinale)*
USED TO TREAT: Constipation (page 221)
SIDE EFFECTS: Burning in mouth, diarrhea, nausea
PRECAUTION: Generally a safe herb

Rosemary *(Rosmarinus officinalis)*
USED TO TREAT: Burning feet (page 250)
SIDE EFFECTS: Diarrhea, kidney irritation, nausea
PRECAUTION: Generally a safe herb

Sage *(Salvia officinalis)*
USED TO TREAT: Diabetes (page 243)
SIDE EFFECTS: Swollen lips and mouth
PRECAUTION: Generally a safe herb

Saw palmetto *(Serenoa repens)*
USED TO TREAT: Prostate cancer (page 186)
SIDE EFFECTS: None known
PRECAUTION: Generally a safe herb

Skullcap *(Scutellaria lateriflora)*
USED TO TREAT: Anxiety (page 159)
SIDE EFFECTS: Confusion, convulsions, giddiness
PRECAUTION: Generally a safe herb

Southernwood *(Artemisia abrotanum)*
USED TO TREAT: Hair loss (page 268)
SIDE EFFECTS: Skin irritation
PRECAUTION: Avoid during pregnancy

St. John's wort *(Hypericum perforatum)*
USED TO TREAT: Depression (page 236)
SIDE EFFECTS: Headache
PRECAUTION: This herb should not be used in combination with certain drugs or foods (see pages 238 and 239 for more information)

Stinging nettle *(Urtica dioica)*
USED TO TREAT: Anemia (page 148), gout (page 262)
SIDE EFFECTS: Burning skin, stomach irritation, urinary retention
PRECAUTION: Generally a safe herb

Stoneroot *(Collinsonia canadensis)*
USED TO TREAT: Hemorrhoids (page 299)
SIDE EFFECTS: None known
PRECAUTION: Generally a safe herb

Tea tree oil *(Melaleuca alternifolia)*
USED TO TREAT: Warts (page 250)
SIDE EFFECTS: Skin irritation
PRECAUTION: Generally a safe herb

TURMERIC *(Curcuma longa)*
USED TO TREAT: Gallbladder disease (page 256)
SIDE EFFECTS: Fertility problems, stomach upset
PRECAUTION: People with clotting disorders should avoid
this herb

VALERIAN *(Valeriana officinalis)*
USED TO TREAT: Anxiety (page 159), insomnia (page
332)
SIDE EFFECTS: Headache, giddiness, nausea, morning
sleepiness
PRECAUTION: Generally a safe herb

WHITE WILLOW *(Salix alba)*
USED TO TREAT: Osteoarthritis (page 165), rheumatoid
arthritis (page 175)
SIDE EFFECTS: Stomach upset, tinnitus
PRECAUTION: People with ulcers should avoid this herb

WILD CHERRY BARK *(Prunus serotina)*
USED TO TREAT: Pneumonia (page 377)
SIDE EFFECTS: Stomach upset
PRECAUTION: Generally a safe herb

WILD YAM *(D. villosa)*
USED TO TREAT: Osteoporosis (page 358), vaginal dry-
ness (page 387), muscle cramps (page 250)
SIDE EFFECTS: Uterine contractions
PRECAUTION: Avoid during pregnancy

WITCH HAZEL *(Hamamelis virginiana)*
USED TO TREAT: Hemorrhoids (page 299), varicose veins
(page 392)
SIDE EFFECTS: None known
PRECAUTION: Generally a safe herb

WOOD BETONY *(Stachys officinalis)*
USED TO TREAT: Anxiety (page 159), hysterectomy recovery (page 313)

SIDE EFFECTS: Vomiting, uterine contractions
PRECAUTION: Avoid during pregnancy

YARROW *(Achillea millefolium)*
USED TO TREAT: Heart disease (page 283), hypertension (page 304)
SIDE EFFECTS: Brown urine
PRECAUTION: Generally a safe herb

YOHIMBINE *(Corynanthe yohimbé)*
USED TO TREAT: Impotence (page 318)
SIDE EFFECTS: Low blood pressure
PRECAUTION: Men with low blood pressure should not use this herb

CHAPTER 3

৵৵

Vitamins and Supplements:
Moving Beyond a Balanced Diet

Even under the best of circumstances, it can be difficult to get all the vitamins and minerals you need from the foods you eat. But the challenge becomes greater as the years go by, because the body becomes progressively less efficient at extracting nutrients from food. Starting at about age 50, the body's ability to absorb nutrients begins to drop off, increasing the possibility of nutritional deficiencies.

Taking a daily vitamin and mineral supplement can make up for many shortcomings in your diet. Studies have found that older people who take a daily multiple supplement have stronger immune systems and suffer fewer infections than those who do not take a supplement. Supplements can also be used to treat disease once it has taken hold. The specific prescriptive advice offered in Part III explains how supplements can be used in the treatment of a number of ailments and conditions.

But how much is enough? And how much is too much?

To help answer these questions, the federal government has established recommended dietary allowances (RDAs) for essential nutrients, using information provided by the Food and Nutrition Board of the National Academy of Sciences National Research Council. The RDAs vary with age and sex, though in an attempt to simplify matters, a single RDA is used on food labels.

RDAs are based on whether a nutrient is essential for the body's health, and on the amount required to prevent deficiency and disease. RDAs are designed to prevent nutritional disease, not to achieve optimal health. That's why many experts recommend that people take vitamins and minerals at higher, therapeutic levels to prevent or manage various ailments or diseases.

Taking vitamins and nutrition supplements to meet the RDAs is not harmful, but self-diagnosing and taking megadoses of specific vitamins can be. When the body encounters large doses of water-soluble vitamins, the excess that it can't use is simply excreted in the urine. However, fat-soluble vitamins can accumulate in the body and cause potential health problems. There is an appropriate range of vitamin intake, and as the chart at the end of this chapter shows, consuming too little or too much of some nutrients can be dangerous.

Scientists have identified approximately forty different nutrients—including vitamins, essential minerals (needed in relatively large amounts), trace minerals (needed in relatively small amounts), and electrolytes—that are necessary for human health.

Vitamins are organic substances that the body needs to regulate metabolism, assist in biochemical processes, and prevent disease. Most vitamins are catalysts (or cofactors) in chemical reactions in the body. For example, vitamin B5 (pantothenic acid) is a cofactor in a series of chemical reactions that burn carbohydrates. Vitamins are either fat soluble or water soluble. As the name implies, fat-soluble vitamins dissolve in the fat; they can be stored by the body for long periods of time and build up to toxic levels if taken in excess. Water-soluble vitamins cannot be stored and must be consumed every day or two; excess levels are eliminated in the urine.

Minerals are basic elements; they cannot be manufactured or broken down by living systems. However, minerals do combine with vitamins, enzymes, and other substances as part of essential metabolic processes in the body. While the vitamin content of foods is stable, the mineral content is not. The mineral content of a plant varies from region to region and plant to plant due to variations in the mineral content of the soil.

Electrolytes are minerals that allow the transmission of electrical impulses in the body. They also help to balance the flow of water across the cell membranes, and they are essential to the maintenance of the balance of water in the body.

What Are Antioxidants?

Oxygen is essential to life. But at the wrong place at the wrong time, oxygen can damage cells, cause cancer, and contribute to aging through a process known as oxidation. As oxygen makes its way through the body, many of its molecules lose an electron, making them chemically unstable. These ions or free radicals are highly reactive; they strive for stability and ultimately "steal" an electron from another molecule, leaving a damaged molecule in their wake. This oxidative damage can cause changes to DNA, leading to cancer, as well as atherosclerosis, cataracts, arthritis, and many other health problems.

Antioxidants minimize the damage of free radicals by freely donating extra electrons, neutralizing the oxygen molecules before they hurt other cells in the body. Antioxidants include the well-known beta-carotene and vitamins A, C, and E, as well as the less famous quercetin, coenzyme Q-10, and lutein among others. Antioxidants are found in many of the foods we eat, as well as in nutrition supplements.

The link between antioxidants and reduced cancer risk is undeniable—though it is not fully understood. Literally hundreds of studies have shown that people who eat large amounts of fresh fruits and vegetables are much less likely to develop cancer than those who do not. What is not known is exactly how the antioxidants perform this task, or whether some other factor is at work. Fruits and vegetables contain antioxidants, as well as other compounds and nutrients that may also play a critical role in disease prevention, either on their own or in combination. For this reason, if you want to hedge your bets against cancer and other diseases associated with aging, consume a wholesome diet rich in fruits and vegetables. While there are conflicting data about the efficacy of antioxidant supplements, many experts recommend taking them as well.

Nutrition as Medicine

If food is good medicine, then so are nutrition supplements. While the best way to get your daily intake of necessary vitamins and minerals is to eat a variety of healthy foods, taking a daily vitamin supplement can also help.

At higher doses, vitamins and minerals can be used to help prevent and cure various illnesses. However, keep in mind that once supplements are taken at therapeutic doses, they are being used as drugs, and they should be granted the same respect as other drugs. In general, unsafe dosages start at about three times the RDA for minerals, five times the RDA for fat-soluble vitamins, and ten times the RDA for water-soluble vitamins.

As is true of other drugs, regular use of vitamin and mineral supplements can become pricey. When shopping for supplements, consider the following tips:

- Look for store brands. All vitamins are essentially the same, so forget the brand names and look for the bargain. If you buy a heavily advertised product, all you're doing is paying for the advertising.
- For the most part, don't worry about going "natural." The body uses both natural and synthetic vitamins in the same way. The big difference is cost: It would take tons of food to extract all the vitamins used in nutrition supplements. Supplements produced in the laboratory are chemically identical—and much cheaper.

One exception: vitamin E. Natural vitamin E is absorbed better than the synthetic version.

- Check the expiration date. Nutrition supplements lose potency over time. Also, be sure to store them in a cool, dry place.
- Don't pay more for "chelated" minerals. Some manufacturers sell supplements that they claim can be absorbed by the body more easily because the minerals have been chelated, or attached to an amino acid. There is no evidence to support this claim—although chelated minerals do cost more, of course.

Finding a Qualified Nutritionist

If you have special nutritional needs, or want help in designing a regimen of nutrition supplements to help manage your specific health needs, you may want to consult a nutrition counselor. For information on finding a qualified nutritionist, contact:

American Association of Nutritional Consultants
880 Canarios Court, Suite 210
Chula Vista, CA 91910-7810
(619) 482-8533

American Academy of Nutrition
3408 Sausalito Drive
Corona Del Mar, CA 92625
(800) 290-4226

American College of Nutrition
722 Robert E. Lee Drive
Wilmington, NC 28412
(919) 452-1222

Consumer Nutrition Hotline
(sponsored by The American Dietetic Association)
(800) 366-1655

The Hotline staff can answer questions and provide free referrals to registered dietitians in your area.

Publications on nutrition are available (some for a fee) from:

American Institute of Nutrition
9650 Rockville Pike, Suite L4500
Bethesda, MD 20814-3990
(301) 530-7050

American Council on Science and Health
1995 Broadway, 16th Floor
New York, NY 10023-5860
(212) 362-7044

The Nutrition Action Health Letter
Center for Science in the Public Interest
1875 Connecticut Avenue, N.W., Suite 300
Washington, DC 20009-5728
(202) 332-9111

Society for Nutrition Education
2001 Killebrew Drive, Suite 340
Minneapolis, MN 55425-1882
(612) 854-0035

Vegetarian Resource Group
P.O. Box 1463
Baltimore, MD 21203
(410) 366-8343

༂

Vitamins, Minerals, and Healing

The following table summarizes the role that key vitamins and minerals play in the body and in the treatment of certain ailments.

<u>VITAMINS</u>

Water-Soluble Vitamins

Vitamin B1 (Thiamin)

WHAT IT DOES: Necessary for carbohydrate metabolism; promotes normal appetite and digestion; needed for nerve function

GOOD FOOD SOURCES: Pork, poultry, liver, pasta, wheat germ, whole-grain or enriched breads, lima beans, seafood, nuts, seeds

SIGNS OF DEFICIENCY: Anxiety, hysteria, nausea, memory loss, irritability, depression, muscle cramps, loss of appetite; in extreme cases, beriberi, paralysis, and heart failure

SIGNS OF OVERDOSE: Unknown; however, due to the interdependency of the B-complex vitamins, an excess of one may cause a deficiency of another

RDA: 1 milligram for women, 1.4 milligrams for men, 1.5 milligrams for pregnant and lactating women

THERAPEUTIC DOSE: 5 milligrams

USED TO TREAT: Vitamin B1 deficiency

WARNING: Antibiotics, sulfa drugs, and oral contraceptives may decrease thiamin levels in the body; eating a high-carbohydrate diet may increase the need for thiamin

Vitamin B2 (Riboflavin)

WHAT IT DOES: Assists in the metabolism of carbohydrates, proteins, and fats; maintains good vision

GOOD FOOD SOURCES: Milk, cheese, fish, eggs, green leafy vegetables, liver, meat, whole-grain or enriched breads and cereals, bee pollen, nuts, wheat germ

SIGNS OF DEFICIENCY: Lesions around the nose and eyes; sores on the lips, mouth, and tongue; intolerance of light

SIGNS OF OVERDOSE: Same as for vitamin B1

RDA: 1.3 milligrams for women, 1.8 milligrams for men, 2 milligrams for pregnant and lactating women

THERAPEUTIC DOSE: 5 milligrams

USED TO TREAT: Vitamin B2 deficiency

WARNING: Using oral contraceptives and exercising strenuously increases the need for riboflavin

VITAMIN B3 (NIACIN)

WHAT IT DOES: Promotes normal appetite and digestion; needed for general metabolism

GOOD FOOD SOURCES: Liver, meat, fish, poultry, green vegetables, nuts, whole-grain or enriched breads and cereals (except corn)

SIGNS OF DEFICIENCY: Irritability, memory loss, headaches, skin disorders

SIGNS OF OVERDOSE: Ulcers, liver disorders, high blood sugar levels, high uric acid levels, depression

RDA: 15 milligrams for women, 18 milligrams for men and pregnant and lactating women

THERAPEUTIC DOSE: 50 milligrams (under a doctor's supervision)

USED TO TREAT: Arthritis, heart disease

WARNING: Niacin should not be used in large amounts by people suffering from gout, peptic ulcers, glaucoma, liver disease, or diabetes

VITAMIN B5 (PANTOTHENIC ACID)

WHAT IT DOES: Needed for the metabolism of carbohydrates, fats, and proteins; also needed for the formation of certain hormones

GOOD FOOD SOURCES: Found in most animal and plant foods; also produced by intestinal bacteria

SIGNS OF DEFICIENCY: Fatigue, numbness, emotional swings

SIGNS OF OVERDOSE: May increase the need for thiamin and lead to thiamin deficiency

RDA: 5 to 10 milligrams (no formal RDAs)

THERAPEUTIC DOSE: 10 milligrams

USED TO TREAT: Vitamin B5 deficiency

VITAMIN B6 (PYRIDOXINE)

WHAT IT DOES: Assists in the metabolism of proteins, carbohydrates, and fats; also aids in the formation of red blood cells and functioning of the nervous system and brain

GOOD FOOD SOURCES: Green leafy vegetables, meat, fish, poultry, whole-grain cereals, liver, nuts, seeds, bananas, avocados, potatoes

SIGNS OF DEFICIENCY: Depression, confusion, convulsions, irritability, insomnia, reduced resistance to infection, sores in the mouth, itchy skin

SIGNS OF OVERDOSE: Overdose can lead to dependency and cause signs of deficiency when intake is reduced to normal levels

RDA: 2 milligrams for women, 2.2 milligrams for men, 2.5 milligrams for pregnant and lactating women

THERAPEUTIC DOSE: 50 milligrams as part of a B-complex supplement

USED TO TREAT: Glaucoma

WARNING: Antidepressants, estrogen, and oral contraceptives may increase the need for vitamin B6

VITAMIN B12 (CYANOCOBALAMINE)

WHAT IT DOES: Necessary for the formation of genetic material and red blood cells

GOOD FOOD SOURCES: Milk, saltwater fish, oysters, meat, liver, kidneys, eggs, pork, cheese, yogurt

SIGNS OF DEFICIENCY: Pernicious anemia

SIGNS OF OVERDOSE: Same as for Vitamin B1

RDA: 3 micrograms for adults, 4 micrograms for pregnant and lactating women

THERAPEUTIC DOSE: 10 micrograms

USED TO TREAT: Alzheimer's disease, dementia, anemia

WARNING: Antigout medications, anticoagulant drugs, and potassium supplements may block the absorption of vitamin B12

VITAMIN H (BIOTIN)

WHAT IT DOES: Involved in the formation of certain fatty acids and in the metabolism of carbohydrates and fats

GOOD FOOD SOURCES: Eggs, green leafy vegetables, liver, string beans, milk, meat, nuts

SIGNS OF DEFICIENCY: Depression, insomnia, muscle pain, anemia (rare except in infants)

SIGNS OF OVERDOSE: Same as for vitamin B1

RDA: 100 to 200 micrograms (no formal RDAs)

THERAPEUTIC DOSE: 200 micrograms

USED TO TREAT: Vitamin H deficiency

WARNING: Consuming saccharin can inhibit biotin absorption

FOLIC ACID (FOLATE)

WHAT IT DOES: Assists in the formation of certain proteins and genetic materials, as well as in the formation of red blood cells

GOOD FOOD SOURCES: Green leafy vegetables, liver, kidney, avocados, wheat germ, legumes, bran, nuts

SIGNS OF DEFICIENCY: Impaired cell division, creation of abnormal red blood cells, anemia, mental problems

SIGNS OF OVERDOSE: Could mask a B12 deficiency

RDA: 400 micrograms, 500 micrograms for pregnant women

THERAPEUTIC DOSE: 400 micrograms

USED TO TREAT: Cancer, heart disease

WARNING: Use of oral contraceptives may increase the need

for folic acid; inadequate intake during pregnancy increases the risk of spina bifida

Vitamin C (Ascorbic Acid)

WHAT IT DOES: Helps bind cells together and strengthen the walls of the blood vessels; helps fight infection; promotes wound healing

GOOD FOOD SOURCES: Citrus fruits and juices, green leafy vegetables, tomatoes, melons, cauliflower, strawberries, new potatoes

SIGNS OF DEFICIENCY: Scurvy, bleeding gums, loose teeth, slow healing, dry and rough skin, loss of appetite

SIGNS OF OVERDOSE: Bladder and kidney stones, urinary tract irritation, diarrhea; overconsumption can lead to dependency, which can cause deficiency symptoms when intake is reduced to normal levels

RDA: 60 milligrams, 100 milligrams for pregnant and lactating women

THERAPEUTIC DOSE: 1,000 to 3,000 milligrams

USED TO TREAT: Alzheimer's disease, anemia, arthritis, bedsores, bronchitis, cancer, cataracts, colds, depression, flu, gallbladder disease, glaucoma, hair loss, heart disease, hypertension, impotence, Parkinson's disease, periodontal disease, pneumonia, tetanus, varicose veins

WARNING: Aspirin, alcohol, analgesics, antidepressants, anticoagulants, oral contraceptives, and steroids may reduce vitamin C levels in the body

Fat-Soluble Vitamins

Vitamin A

WHAT IT DOES: Helps to form and maintain healthy function of the eyes, hair, teeth, gums, and mucous membranes; also involved in fat metabolism. Vitamin A in animal tissues is called retinol; vitamin A in plants is called beta-carotene. (Beta-carotene is sometimes called a provitamin because it must be broken down by the body into vitamin A before it acts as a vitamin.) Both vitamin A and beta-carotene are antioxidants, which may help protect against cancer and improve resistance to certain diseases.

GOOD FOOD SOURCES: Whole milk, butter, fortified margarine, eggs, green leafy and yellow vegetables and fruits, organ meats, cheese, and fish

SIGNS OF DEFICIENCY: Night blindness, retarded growth, impaired resistance to disease, infection, rough skin, dry eyes

SIGNS OF OVERDOSE: Headaches, blurred vision, skin rash, extreme fatigue, diarrhea, nausea, loss of appetite, hair loss, menstrual irregularities, liver damage, dizziness

RDA: 5,000 IU

THERAPEUTIC DOSE: 5,000 to 10,000 IU

USED TO TREAT: Arthritis, bronchitis, cataracts, colds, heart disease, impotence, pneumonia, tetanus

WARNING: Vitamin A should not be taken in large amounts by pregnant women or people suffering from liver disease, diabetics, and by those with hypothyroidism

Vitamin D

WHAT IT DOES: Needed for the body to absorb and metabolize calcium and phosphorus to build bones and teeth

GOOD FOOD SOURCES: Fortified milk, liver, fish liver and fish oils, egg yolks, butter; exposure to the sun's ultraviolet rays enables the body to produce its own Vitamin D

SIGNS OF DEFICIENCY: Rickets in children; thin bones in adults

SIGNS OF OVERDOSE: Calcium deposits in the body, nausea, loss of appetite, kidney stones, high blood pressure, high cholesterol levels, fragile bones

RDA: 5 micrograms for men, 10 micrograms for women, 15 micrograms for pregnant and lactating women

THERAPEUTIC DOSE: 10 micrograms

USED TO TREAT: Glaucoma

WARNING: Vitamin D should not be taken without calcium;

intestinal disorders, liver problems, and gallbladder disease can interfere with the absorption of vitamin D

Vitamin E

WHAT IT DOES: Helps the body form red blood cells, muscles and other tissues; necessary for the breakdown of fats

GOOD FOOD SOURCES: Wheat germ, vegetable oils, margarine, nuts, seeds, eggs, milk, whole-grain cereals, breads

SIGNS OF DEFICIENCY: Deficiency is rare except in people with an impaired absorption of fat

SIGNS OF OVERDOSE: Not clearly understood

RDA: 30 IU

THERAPEUTIC DOSE: 400 to 800 IU

USED TO TREAT: Alzheimer's disease, arthritis, bedsores, cancer, cataracts, constipation, diabetes, heart disease, hysterectomy (recovery), menopausal symptoms, obesity, periodontal disease, vaginal dryness, varicose veins

WARNING: People with diabetes, thyroid disease, or heart disease should not take high doses of vitamin E

Vitamin K

WHAT IT DOES: Needed for normal blood clotting and bone metabolism

GOOD FOOD SOURCES: Green leafy vegetables, peas, cereals, dairy products, liver, potatoes, cabbage, wheat germ, tomatoes, eggs; also produced by intestinal bacteria

SIGNS OF DEFICIENCY: Bleeding disorders and liver damage

SIGNS OF OVERDOSE: Jaundice in infants

RDA: 70 to 140 micrograms (formal RDAs not established)

THERAPEUTIC DOSE: Not recommended due to its toxicity

WARNING: Antibiotics can interfere with the absorption of vitamin K

MINERALS

ESSENTIAL MINERALS

CALCIUM

WHAT IT DOES: Helps build strong bones and teeth; helps blood clot; helps nerve and muscle function. Recent research indicates that calcium supplements can reduce the risk of high blood pressure in pregnant women.

GOOD FOOD SOURCES: Milk and milk products, cheese, green leafy vegetables, citrus fruits, dried peas and beans, sardines (with bones), shellfish, whole-grain breads

SIGNS OF DEFICIENCY: Rickets in children; osteoporosis in adults

SIGNS OF OVERDOSE: Drowsiness, calcium deposits, impaired absorption of iron and other minerals

RDA: 800 milligrams for men, 1,200 milligrams for women, 1,500 milligrams for pregnant and lactating women

THERAPEUTIC DOSE: 1,500 milligrams

USED TO TREAT: Anxiety, dental problems, depression, glaucoma, heart disease, hypertension, insomnia, osteoporosis, Parkinson's disease, periodontal disease

WARNING: People with kidney stones or kidney disease should not take calcium supplements; too much calcium can interfere with absorption of zinc

PHOSPHORUS

WHAT IT DOES: Helps build bones and teeth; needed to change food into energy

GOOD FOOD SOURCES: Meat, poultry, fish, eggs, dried peas and beans, milk and milk products, egg yolk, phosphates in processed foods and soft drinks

SIGNS OF DEFICIENCY: Weakness, bone pain, decreased appetite, anemia

SIGNS OF OVERDOSE: Upset in calcium-phosphorus ratio, hindering uptake of calcium

RDA: 800 milligrams for adults, 1,200 milligrams for pregnant and lactating women

THERAPEUTIC DOSE: 800 milligrams

USED TO TREAT: Phosphorus deficiency

WARNING: Excess phosphorus can interfere with calcium uptake

MAGNESIUM

WHAT IT DOES: Necessary for the metabolism of protein and carbohydrates

GOOD FOOD SOURCES: Raw leafy green vegetables, nuts, soy beans, whole-grain breads and cereals, shrimp

SIGNS OF DEFICIENCY: Muscle tremors, leg cramps, weakness, irregular heartbeat, constipation

SIGNS OF OVERDOSE: Upset in calcium-magnesium ratio, resulting in impaired nervous system function; especially dangerous in people with impaired kidney function

RDA: 300 milligrams for women, 350 milligrams for men, 450 milligrams for pregnant and lactating women

THERAPEUTIC DOSE: 750 milligrams

USED TO TREAT: Angina, anxiety, dental problems, depression, diabetes, heart disease, hypertension, hysterectomy (recovery), insomnia, osteoporosis, Parkinson's disease, periodontal disease

WARNING: Consumption of alcohol, diuretics, and high amounts of zinc and vitamin D all increase the body's need for magnesium

IODINE

WHAT IT DOES: Necessary for the normal function of the thyroid gland

GOOD FOOD SOURCES: Iodized salt, seafood, fish liver oil

SIGNS OF DEFICIENCY: Thyroid enlargement

SIGNS OF OVERDOSE: Poisoning

RDA: 150 micrograms for adults, 200 micrograms for pregnant and lactating women

THERAPEUTIC DOSE: 50 to 300 micrograms

USED TO TREAT: Iodine deficiency

WARNING: People with hypothyroid disorder should avoid high-iodine foods; when taken in large amounts some raw foods (Brussels sprouts, cabbage, kale, peaches, spinach) can block the uptake of iodine into the thyroid

IRON

WHAT IT DOES: Combines with protein to make hemoglobin (which carries oxygen in the blood) and myoglobin (which stores oxygen in the muscles)

GOOD FOOD SOURCES: Liver, red meat, egg yolks, shellfish, green leafy vegetables, peas, beans, dried prunes, raisins, apricots, whole-grain and enriched breads and cereals, nuts

SIGNS OF DEFICIENCY: Anemia, weakness, fatigue, headache, shortness of breath

SIGNS OF OVERDOSE: Buildup in the liver, pancreas, and heart

RDA: 10 milligrams for men, 12 milligrams for women, 15 milligrams for pregnant and lactating women

THERAPEUTIC DOSE: 18 milligrams

USED TO TREAT: Anemia

WARNING: High amounts of zinc and vitamin E can interfere with iron absorption; tannins (found in tea) can also inhibit iron absorption

ZINC

WHAT IT DOES: Necessary for the red blood cells to move carbon dioxide away from the tissues; involved in the metabolism of carbohydrates and vitamins

GOOD FOOD SOURCES: Meats, fish, egg yolks, milk, oysters, whole grains, nuts, legumes

SIGNS OF DEFICIENCY: Loss of taste, delayed wound healing, infertility

SIGNS OF OVERDOSE: Nausea, vomiting, abdominal pain

RDA: 15 milligrams for adults, 25 milligrams for pregnant and lactating women

THERAPEUTIC DOSE: 50 milligrams

USED TO TREAT: Alzheimer's disease, arthritis, bedsores, bronchitis, colds, dental problems, hemorrhoids, impotence, osteoporosis, periodontal disease, pneumonia, tetanus

WARNING: Drinking "hard" (mineral-laden) water can upset zinc levels

IMPORTANT TRACE MINERALS

CHROMIUM

WHAT IT DOES: Necessary for blood-sugar regulation

GOOD FOOD SOURCES: Brewer's yeast, oysters, eggs, whole grains

SIGNS OF DEFICIENCY: Infertility, cloudy corneas, atherosclerosis

SIGNS OF OVERDOSE: Chronic exposure to chromium dust in industry has been linked to lung cancer

RDA: 50 to 200 micrograms

THERAPEUTIC DOSE: 200 micrograms (under doctor's supervision)

USED TO TREAT: Diabetes

COPPER

WHAT IT DOES: Necessary for maintenance of healthy blood cells and bones

GOOD FOOD SOURCES: Liver, kidney, nuts, shellfish, legumes, yeast, cocoa, whole-grain cereals

SIGNS OF DEFICIENCY: Anemia, elevated cholesterol levels, infertility

SIGNS OF OVERDOSE: Nausea, vomiting, muscle aches, stomach pains

RDA: 2 milligrams

THERAPEUTIC DOSE: 2.5 milligrams

USED TO TREAT: Copper deficiency

WARNING: High levels of zinc and vitamin C can reduce copper levels

FLUORIDE

WHAT IT DOES: Necessary for strong bones and teeth

GOOD FOOD SOURCES: China tea, seafood, wheat, carrots, currants

SIGNS OF DEFICIENCY: Tooth decay

SIGNS OF OVERDOSE: Discolored teeth

RDA: Nutritional requirements unknown; the average daily intake ranges from 0.5 to 1.5 milligrams in areas with unfluoridated water and from 2 to 4 milligrams per day in areas with a fluoridated water supply

THERAPEUTIC DOSE: 1 milligram; consult doctor or dentist

USED TO TREAT: Tooth decay, osteoporosis

MANGANESE

WHAT IT DOES: Necessary for tendons and bone formation, nervous system function, and fat and vitamin metabolism

GOOD FOOD SOURCES: Bran, coffee, tea, nuts, beans, peas

SIGNS OF DEFICIENCY: Cartilage problems, infertility, birth defects

SIGNS OF OVERDOSE: Irritability, muscle tremors

RDA: 2.5 to 5 milligrams (not a formal RDA)

THERAPEUTIC DOSE: The amount in most vitamin/mineral supplements should be sufficient

SELENIUM

WHAT IT DOES: Works with vitamin E in the breakdown of fat in the body; necessary for healthy liver, heart, and white blood cells

GOOD FOOD SOURCES: Seafood, egg yolks, chicken, meat, garlic, whole-grain cereals, brewer's yeast, fish, organ meats

SIGNS OF DEFICIENCY: Liver disease, skin problems, arthritis

SIGNS OF OVERDOSE: Unknown

RDA: 50 to 200 micrograms (not a formal RDA)

THERAPEUTIC DOSE: 200 micrograms

USED TO TREAT: Anxiety, arthritis, cancer, cataracts

Electrolytes

Sodium

WHAT IT DOES: Helps maintain water balance inside and outside the cells; involved in nerve and muscle function

GOOD FOOD SOURCES: Salt, processed foods, ham, meat, fish, poultry, eggs, milk, salted crackers

SIGNS OF DEFICIENCY: Water retention, muscle cramps, headache, weakness, exhaustion, nausea

SIGNS OF OVERDOSE: High blood pressure, kidney disease, congestive heart failure

RDA: 300 milligrams

THERAPEUTIC DOSE: 300 milligrams

USED TO TREAT: Sodium deficiency

WARNING: High sodium levels may result in potassium deficiency and liver and kidney disease

Potassium

WHAT IT DOES: With sodium, it helps regulate fluid balance in the body; also needed for the transmission of nerve impulses, muscle contractions, and metabolism

GOOD FOOD SOURCES: Bananas, dried fruits, peanut butter, potatoes, orange juice, fruits and vegetables, milk, beef

SIGNS OF DEFICIENCY: Muscle weakness, irritability, irregular heartbeat, kidney and lung failure

SIGNS OF OVERDOSE: Cardiac irregularities

RDA: 900 milligrams

THERAPEUTIC DOSE: 5 grams

USED TO TREAT: Heart disease

WARNING: Use of diuretics and laxatives can reduce potassium levels

CHAPTER 4

❧

Homeopathy:
The Dilution Solution

Homeopathy is based on the premise that less is more. This holistic approach to healing relies on the use of infinitesimal amounts of substances—plants, minerals, chemicals, microorganisms, animal materials, and even modern drugs—to boost the body's defenses against illness.

One of the principle tenets of homeopathy is the law of similars—or "like cures like"—the theory that a remedy taken in small amounts will cure the same symptoms that it would cause if taken in large amounts. In fact, the word *homeopathy* has its roots in the Greek words *homo,* meaning "like, similar" and *pathos,* meaning "suffering or disease."

Consider the medicinal use of belladonna, an extract from the poisonous plant deadly nightshade. If taken internally, belladonna can cause high fever, flushed face, confusion, and other flulike symptoms. However, belladonna is one of the homeopathic remedies for fever and flu pre-

cisely because it causes these symptoms. Of course, the
actual amount of belladonna used in the homeopathic remedy is dramatically diluted. In fact, the active ingredient in
a homeopathic remedy is diluted to such a degree that not
a single molecule of the active ingredient can be found in
the solution in its final form. Despite the dilution, there is
evidence that homeopathic remedies work, as you will see
later in this chapter.

The dependence on dilution illustrates the second law of
homeopathy, the law of infinitesimals. This theory states
that the smaller the dose of an active ingredient, the more
effective the cure. However, for this less-is-more principle
to work, each time the solution is diluted, it must be
"potentized" (or shaken) to create "memory of the energy" that cures the body. The law of infinitesimals was
discovered through careful experimentation by Dr. Samuel
Christian Hahnemann (1755–1843), the founder of the
practice of homeopathy.

A Brief History of Homeopathy

In the early nineteenth century Dr. Hahnemann, a German
physician, grew frustrated by the crude and often dangerous medical practices of his day, including bloodletting and
massive doses of drugs that caused diarrhea and vomiting.
Not surprisingly, these harsh measures often did more
harm than good.

Hahnemann espoused many radical ideas, including the
importance of a balanced diet, regular exercise, fresh air,
and less confined housing. His ideas were not well received; Hahnemann eventually left his medical practice
and became a translator. In 1790, while translating *A Trea-
tise on Materia Medica* by Dr. William Cullen, Hahnemann
encountered a passage about Peruvian bark (cinchona).
Cullen had written that quinine, which was purified from
the bark of the cinchona tree, could be used to treat malaria because of its astringent qualities. Hahnemann, a
chemist by training, was baffled by this statement because

he knew there were many other astringent substances that had no effect whatsoever on malaria. In response, he began to experiment.

First, Hahnemann himself took quinine, only to find that he developed the symptoms of malaria, including fever, chills, thirst, and a pounding headache. Through his observations during a series of experiments—both on himself and on his friends—he developed the homeopathic law of similars. He concluded that the quinine prompted the body to mount its defenses against malaria because the drug caused symptoms similar to those caused by the disease itself.

In further experiments, known as "provings," Hahnemann observed that the substances caused significant side effects when used in high concentrations, but he could dilute the medication and protect the healing powers through "potentization." In fact, his tests led Hahnemann to conclude that by repeatedly diluting a substance with distilled water or alcohol and shaking it vigorously between dilutions, he could actually increase the strength or potency of the medicine. These findings resulted in the law of infinitesimals.

In the nineteenth century Hahnemann's theories were put to the test in dealing with epidemic diseases, such as cholera, typhoid, and yellow fever. Homeopathic remedies were credited with saving many lives, and interest in homeopathy spread across Europe. (Modern critics claim that many conventional nineteenth-century treatments actually increased fluid loss, exacerbating illness and causing dehydration and death. Homeopathic remedies, on the other hand, allowed the illness to run its course without causing further health problems.)

In the United States the first homeopathic college opened in Philadelphia in 1836, and eight years later a group of homeopaths formed the American Institute of Homeopathy, the first national medical organization in the country. Two years later the American Medical Association was formed, in part to stem the tide of defections by conventional physicians to homeopathy. By the end of the century, there were 15,000 homeopaths and 22 schools of homeopathy nationwide.

Homeopathy also flourished and continues to thrive in Europe, particularly in Great Britain, where the Queen of England has her own homeopathic physician and the British National Health Service covers homeopathic procedures. Today more than 40 percent of British, French, and Dutch doctors use homeopathy or refer some patients to homeopaths, as do 20 percent of German physicians.

At the end of the nineteenth century fully one out of every five American doctors practiced homeopathy, but by the middle of the twentieth century the American practice had all but died out. One reason was that professional medical groups often expelled physicians who practiced homeopathy or consulted with homeopaths; another factor was that the discovery of antibiotics and other advances in modern medicine lured people to support a more "scientific" approach to healing.

Today homeopathy is experiencing a comeback. Until recently Americans put their trust in high-tech healing, but in the last decade or so they have grown frustrated with the limitations of conventional medicine and turned back to low-tech, natural treatments for many medical problems. As a result, the two-hundred-year-old practice of homeopathy has once again become a popular option.

Putting Homeopathy to the Test

Even the staunchest supporters of homeopathy must admit that its theories defy many of the laws of physical science as we know them. Skeptics charge that any healing that takes places stems from the placebo effect, the benefit a patient gets just by believing that a particular treatment will work. However, a number of studies published in respected medical journals have shown that homeopathic remedies work. Consider the evidence:

- 1986: Researchers in Scotland gave a homeopathic hay fever remedy to 144 people with a pollen allergy. To eliminate prejudice on the part of the researchers, the study was double-blind and placebo-controlled, meaning that neither the researchers nor the participants knew who was receiving the homeopathic remedy and who was receiving the placebo. Compared with those who took the placebo, the homeopathic group showed a significant reduction in symptoms, and their need for antihistamines dropped by 50 percent.
- 1988: A French allergist (who was not a homeopath) diluted an antibody 120 times, to the point that the final solution contained no measurable amount of the original antibody. But the final solution still had a noticeable effect on white blood cells, just as diluted homeopathic remedies have an effect on illness.
- 1989: Nonhomeopathic researchers in Great Britain conducted a double-blind, placebo-controlled study to test a homeopathic flu remedy on nearly 500 people. After two days the homeopathic remedy had relieved twice as many flu symptoms as the placebo.
- 1990: German researchers tested eight homeopathic remedies on 61 people with varicose veins as part of a double-blind, placebo-controlled study. Among the participants who took the homeopathic remedies, symptoms improved by 44 percent; among those who took the placebo, symptoms became 18 percent worse.
- 1991: A British medical journal published an analysis of 105 clinical studies involving the efficacy of homeopathy. The homeopathic treatment was found to be more effective than a placebo in 81 of the studies. Critics of homeopathy charged that many of the studies were poorly designed, but a review of 26 of the better-controlled studies found that 15 demonstrated the benefit of homeopathic treatments.
- 1994: A study published in the British medical journal *The Lancet* found that homeopathic treatments out-

performed a placebo in bringing relief to 28 patients
allergic to dust mites.
- 1994: The peer-reviewed American medical journal
  Pediatrics reported that among 81 children in Nicara-
  gua treated for diarrhea, those given a homeopathic
  treatment in addition to the standard oral rehydration
  therapy got well faster than those who got the standard treatment alone. Among the children in the control group, the diarrhea lasted an average of four days,
  but in the group receiving the homeopathic treatment,
  it lasted two and a half days.

Despite the mounting evidence, no one really under-
stands exactly how or why homeopathy works. Some researchers have speculated that the "potentization"—the
repeated diluting and shaking of the substances—creates a
distinctive electrochemical pattern in the water. According
to this theory of energy medicine, when a patient takes the
homeopathic remedy, the electrochemical pattern in the
solution somehow subtly changes the electromagnetic
fields in the body.

Not all scientists accept this explanation, and ultimately
the question of how homeopathy works remains open. But
you can take advantage of the healing benefits of homeopathy without understanding all its mysteries. All you need
to do is keep an open mind and learn more about how you
can use homeopathy to manage the ailments associated
with growing older.

Practicing Homeopathy

A visit to a homeopath is nothing like a visit to a conventional physician. Homeopaths and medical doctors approach healing from different points of view. Homeopaths
treat the person, not the disease. They believe that illness
is not localized in one organ or manifested in a single
symptom. When deciding which of the three thousand ho-

meopathic remedies they should prescribe for a patient, they consider the entire person, both mind and body.

In contrast, conventional physicians typically focus on suppressing symptoms, taking little or no account of the person's emotional or overall physical condition. They see their mission as one of lowering fevers, easing aches and pains, and eliminating other symptoms or complaints, rather than treating the person as a whole.

These marked differences in approach show up in the first office visit. While a conventional doctor usually spends less than ten minutes with a patient, a homeopath can spend over an hour interviewing that patient, asking detailed questions about medical history and personal characteristics. The homeopath will construct a patient profile, based on overall energy, sensitivity to temperature, sleep habits, food preferences, emotional state, and other factors that help the homeopath understand the patient and prescribe the best remedy.

The selection of the appropriate homeopathic remedy varies from patient to patient, depending on the patient's individual needs rather than the symptoms. For example, two people might pass a cold virus from one to the other, but each person would receive a different treatment, based on their specific personal needs.

Despite its many benefits, homeopathy is not the best treatment for all illnesses or conditions. It is not appropriate for medical problems that involve physical deformities, tissue damage, or cancer, or for situations that might require surgery. Since it can take a great deal of experience and expertise to determine which homeopathic remedies would work best in a given situation, the remedies outlined in Part III of this book tend to be general. You should limit your home use of homeopathic remedies to the treatment of relatively minor or straightforward ailments. If you try a remedy and fail to find relief, consult a trained homeopath.

Finding the Right Solution

To ensure efficacy and purity, homeopathic remedies are prepared according to standards of the *Homeopathic Pharmacopoeia of the United States*. First, the raw material or active ingredient is dissolved in an alcohol/water mixture that contains about 90 percent pure alcohol and 10 percent distilled water. The mixture then stands for two to four weeks, with periodic shakings. It is then strained, and the resulting liquid is known as the mother tincture.

Homeopathic remedies come in a variety of potencies, based on the number of times they have been diluted. Topical homeopathic creams, ointments, and salves can be made by mixing the tincture with a cream or gel base. The three most common forms of homeopathic remedies are the mother tincture, x potencies, and c potencies.

- The mother tincture. This tincture is an alcohol-based extract of a specific substance. Mother tinctures are usually used topically.
- X potencies. The x represents the Roman numeral 10. In homeopathic remedies with x potencies, the mother tincture has been diluted to one part in ten (one drop of tincture for every nine drops of alcohol/water solution). The number before the x tells how many times the mother tincture has been diluted. For example, a 12x potency represents 12 dilutions of one in ten. The more the substance is diluted, the more potent it becomes, so a remedy with a 30x potency is considered stronger or more potent than one with a 12x potency.
- C potencies. The c represents the Roman numeral 100. Homeopathy remedies with a c potency have been diluted to one part in 100 (one drop of tincture for every 99 drops of alcohol/water solution). Again, the number before the c represents the number of dilutions. A 3c potency represents a substance that has been diluted to one part in 100 three times; by the

time 3c is reached, the dilution is one part per million. In most cases, 6c is the potency recommended for acute or self-limiting ailments, and 30c for chronic conditions or emergencies.

The 30c potency should not be administered for more than four doses without a clear and definite result. If your condition improves after four doses, wait and see what happens. If the symptoms return, take up to four more doses, then wait again. If you experience no improvement after four doses, discontinue the treatment and try something else, or contact a qualified homeopath.

Homeopathic remedies come in pellet, tablet, and liquid forms. The pellets and tablets consist primarily of sugar. (They actually contain milk sugar, or lactose, so people with lactose intolerance should use a liquid form.) When taking homeopathic pellets or tablets, avoid touching them. Instead, shake the pellets into a measuring spoon and place them in your mouth to allow them to dissolve. Unless otherwise noted, a dose is one tablet, one drop, or just enough pellets to cover the area of the small fingernail.

When taking a homeopathic remedy, do not eat for at least a half hour before or afterward. Strong flavors can decrease the effectiveness of the remedies. Likewise, avoid strong odors, which can also affect the efficacy of the treatment.

If you are using an appropriate homeopathic remedy, it should work quickly, and then you can discontinue treatment. Although negative reactions to homeopathic remedies are rare, they can happen. If your condition gets worse after taking a particular remedy, stop taking it. Wait for the aggravation to subside and then try it again. If the problems resurface, stop using the remedy and seek help from a professional homeopath.

Homeopathic remedies will not interfere with any drugs your doctor prescribes for you. However, many conventional drugs—including steroids, tranquilizers, oral contraceptives, sleeping pills, and antihistamines—can modify or completely block the effects of homeopathic drugs. Discuss any drug reactions with your doctor. Do not stop taking any drugs—especially prescription drugs—without first consulting your doctor.

How to Find a Qualified Homeopath

Homeopathy is considered a practice of medicine, and it can be performed legally only by medical professionals. The requirements for licensure vary from state to state. While medical doctors (M.D.'s) and osteopaths (D.O.'s) can practice homeopathy in all states, many other medical professionals—such as naturopaths (N.D.'s), and chiropractors (D.C.'s)—may be qualified to practice homeopathy, provided they meet the necessary licensing requirements.

For an information packet on homeopathy and a directory of practitioners, contact:

National Center for Homeopathy
801 N. Fairfax Street, Suite 306
Alexandria, VA 22314
(703) 548-7790
There is a $6 fee for the information packet and directory. The Center also publishes the monthly magazine *Homeopathy Today* as well as other books and products.

International Foundation for Homeopathy
P.O. Box 7
Edmons, WA 98020
(206) 776-4147
There is a $4 fee for the information packet and directory.

Homeopathic Educational Services
2124 Kittredge Street
Berkeley, CA 94704

You may also want to buy homeopathic remedies for home treatment of many common ailments. The following manufacturers supply homeopathic remedies by mail:

The Apothecary
5415 Cedar Lane
Bethesda, MD 20814
(301) 530-0800

Apthorp Pharmacy
2201 Broadway at 78th Street
New York, NY 10024
(800) 775-3582
(212) 877-3480

Bailey's Pharmacy
175 Harvard Avenue
Allston, MA 02134
(800) 239-6206
(617) 782-7202

Budget Pharmacy
3001 N.W. 7th Street
Miami, FL 33125
(800) 221-9772

Boericke and Tafel
2381 Circadian Way
Santa Rosa, CA 95407
(707) 571-8202

Dolisos America
3014 Rigel Avenue
Las Vegas, NV 89102
(702) 871-7153

Five Elements Center
115 Route 46W
Building D, Suite 29
Mt. Lakes, NJ 07046
(201) 402-8510

Hahnemann Pharmacy
828 San Pablo Avenue
Albany, CA 94706
(510) 527-3003

Homeopathic Educational Services
2124 Kittredge Street
Berkeley, CA 94704
(510) 649-0294

Homeopathy Overnight
4111 Simon Road
Youngstown, OH 44512
(800) ARNICA-30

Humphreys Pharmacal Co.
63 Meadow Road
Rutherford, NJ 07070
(201) 933-7744

Luyties Pharmacal Co.
4200 Laclede Avenue
St. Louis, MO 63108
(800) 325-8080

Santa Monica Homeopathic Co.
629 Broadway
Santa Monica, CA 90401
(310) 395-1131

Standard Homeopathy Co.
P.O. Box 61067
154 W. 131st Street
Los Angeles, CA 90061
(213) 321-4284

Taylor's Pharmacy
230 North Park Avenue
Winter Park, FL 32789
(407) 644-1025

Washington Homeopathic Pharmacy
4914 Del Ray Avenue
Bethesda, MD 20814
(301) 656-1695

Weleda Pharmacy
175 North Route 9W
Congers, NY 10920
(914) 268-8572

HOMEOPATHIC REMEDIES FOR COMMON AILMENTS

The following homeopathic remedies are used to treat the medical conditions covered in this book. This list can be used as a cross-reference with the conditions listed in Part III. It also provides both the common abbreviations and the full Latin name for each of the remedies, to avoid confusion when purchasing products.

ACONITE. *(Aconitum napellus)*
SOURCE: Wolfsbane, blue aconite
USED TO TREAT: Bronchitis (page 213), colds (page 213), heart disease (page 283), insomnia (page 332), rheumatoid arthritis (page 175)

AESCULUS *(Aesculus hippocastanum)*
SOURCE: Horse chestnut
USED TO TREAT: Hemorrhoids (page 299)

AGNUS *(Agnus castus)*
SOURCE: Chaste tree
USED TO TREAT: Impotence (page 318)

AGARICUS *(Agaricus muscarius)*
SOURCE: Fly agaric
USED TO TREAT: Parkinson's disease (page 366)

ALLIUM *(Allium cepa)*
SOURCE: Red onion
USED TO TREAT: Bronchitis (page 213), colds (page 213)

ALUMINA *(Alumina)*
SOURCE: Aluminum oxide
USED TO TREAT: Alzheimer's disease (page 139), constipation (page 221), dementia (page 139)

AMYL *(Amyl nitrite)*
SOURCE: Amyl nitrite
USED TO TREAT: Menopausal symptoms (page 340)

APIS *(Apis mellifica)*
SOURCE: Honey bee (whole bee or venom)
USED TO TREAT: Foot ache (page 250)

ARGENTUM NIT. *(Argentum nitricum)*
SOURCE: Silver nitrate
USED TO TREAT: Diabetes (page 243)

ARNICA *(Arnica montana)*
SOURCE: Leopard's bane, Fallkraut
USED TO TREAT: Foot ache (page 250), osteoarthritis (page 165), gout (page 262), heart disease (page 283), osteoporosis (page 358), toothache (page 228); also following breast cancer surgery and hysterectomy (pages 186, 313)

ARSENICUM *(Arsenicum album)*
SOURCE: Arsenic trioxide
USED TO TREAT: Anxiety (page 159), flu (page 213)

ARSENICUM IOD. *(Arsenicum iodatum)*
SOURCE: Arsenic iodide
USED TO TREAT: Heart disease (page 283)

AURUM *(Aurum metallicum)*
SOURCE: Gold
USED TO TREAT: Depression (page 236)

BARYTA CARB. *(Baryta carbonica)*
SOURCE: Barium carbonate
USED TO TREAT: Hair loss (page 268), heart disease (page 283), hypertension (page 304)

BELLADONNA *(Atropa belladonna)*
SOURCE: Deadly nightshade
USED TO TREAT: Gallstones (page 256), toothache (page 228)

BERBERIS *(Berberis vulgaris)*
SOURCE: Common barberry
USED TO TREAT: Gallstones (page 256)

BRYONIA *(Bryonia alba)*
SOURCE: White bryony
USED TO TREAT: Constipation (page 221), osteoarthritis (page 165), menopausal symptoms (page 340), pneumonia (page 377), vaginal dryness (page 387)

CACTUS *(Cactus grandiflourus)*
SOURCE: Night-blooming cereus
USED TO TREAT: Angina (page 154)

CALCAREA *(Calcarea carbonica)*
SOURCE: Calcium carbonate
USED TO TREAT: Anxiety (page 159), cataracts (page 205), menopausal symptoms (page 340), obesity (page 352)

CALCAREA PHOS. *(Calcarea phosphorica)*
SOURCE: Calcium phosphate
USED TO TREAT: Osteoarthritis (page 165)

CAPSICUM *(Capsicum annuum)*
SOURCE: Cayenne pepper
USED TO TREAT: Hemorrhoids (page 299), obesity (page 352)

CAUSTICUM *(Causticum Hahnemanni)*
SOURCE: Potassium hydrate
USED TO TREAT: Incontinence (page 324)

CHAMOMILLA *(Chamomilla vulgaris)*
SOURCE: German chamomile

USED TO TREAT: Broken, cracked, or chipped teeth (page 228); toothache (page 228)

CHENOPODIUM *(Chenopodium anthelminticum)*
SOURCE: Jerusalem oat
USED TO TREAT: Hearing loss (page 274)

CHINA *(China officinalis)*
SOURCE: Peruvian bark, quinine
USED TO TREAT: Anemia (page 148), gallstones (page 256), hearing loss (page 274)

COFFEA *(Coffea cruda)*
SOURCE: Unroasted coffee
USED TO TREAT: Insomnia (page 332), toothache (page 228)

COLCHICUM *(Colchicum autumnale)*
SOURCE: Meadow saffron
USED TO TREAT: Gout (page 262)

CONIUM *(Conium maculatum)*
SOURCE: Hemlock
USED TO TREAT: Impotence (page 318)

DIGITALIS *(Digitalis purpurea)*
SOURCE: Red foxglove
USED TO TREAT: Heart disease (page 283)

EUPATORIUM *(Eupatorium perfoliatum)*
SOURCE: Boneset
USED TO TREAT: Flu (page 213)

EUPHRASIA *(Euphrasia officinalis)*
SOURCE: Common eyebright
USED TO TREAT: Bronchitis (page 213), colds (page 213)

FERRUM *(Ferrum metallicum)*
SOURCE: Iron
USED TO TREAT: Anemia (page 148), obesity (page 352)

FERRUM PHOS. *(Ferrum phosphoricum)*
SOURCE: Iron phosphate
USED TO TREAT: Flu (page 213), incontinence (page 324)

GELSEMIUM *(Gelsemium sempervirens)*
SOURCE: Yellow jasmine
USED TO TREAT: Bronchitis (page 213), colds (page 213)

GLONOINUM *(Glonoinum)*
SOURCE: Trinitroglycerine
USED TO TREAT: Angina (page 154)

GRAPHITES *(Graphites)*
SOURCE: Black pencil lead
USED TO TREAT: Hearing loss (page 274), obesity (page 352)

HAMAMELIS *(Hamamelis virginiana)*
SOURCE: Common witch hazel
USED TO TREAT: Hemorrhoids (page 299), varicose veins (page 392)

HYOSCYAMUS *(Hyoscyamus niger)*
SOURCE: Henbane
USED TO TREAT: Parkinson's disease (page 366)

HYPERICUM *(Hypericum perforatum)*
SOURCE: St. John's wort
USED TO TREAT: Broken, cracked, or chipped teeth (page 228)

IGNATIA *(Ignatia amara)*
SOURCE: St. Ignatius's bean
USED TO TREAT: Anxiety (page 159), depression (page 236), impotence (page 318), insomnia (page 332)

KALI CARB. *(Kali carbonicum)*
SOURCE: Potassium carbonate
USED TO TREAT: Obesity (page 352)

KALI PHOS. *(Kali phosphoricum)*
SOURCE: Potassium phosphate
USED TO TREAT: Periodontal disease (page 371)

KREOSOTUM *(Kreosotum)*
SOURCE: Creosote
USED TO TREAT: Periodontal disease (page 371), tooth decay (page 228)

LACHESIS *(Trigonocephalus lachesis)*
SOURCE: Surucucu snake venom
USED TO TREAT: Heart disease (page 283), menopausal symptoms (page 340)

LATRODECTUS *(Latrodectus mactans)*
SOURCE: American spider
USED TO TREAT: Angina (page 154)

LEDUM *(Ledum palustre)*
SOURCE: Wild rosemary
USED TO TREAT: Gout (page 262), osteoarthritis (page 165)

LILIUM *(Lilium tigrinum)*
SOURCE: Tiger lily
USED TO TREAT: Angina (page 154)

LYCOPODIUM *(Lycopodium clavatum)*
SOURCE: Wolfsclow club moss
USED TO TREAT: Alzheimer's disease (page 139), anxiety (page 159), dementia (page 139), hair loss (page 268), impotence (page 318)

MERCURIUS *(Mercurius solubilis hahnemanni)*
SOURCE: Mercury

USED TO TREAT: Flu (page 213), Parkinson's disease (page 366), tooth decay (page 228)

MERCURIUS CORR. *(Mercurius corrosivus)*
SOURCE: Corrosive sublimate of mercury
USED TO TREAT: Periodontal disease (page 371)

MURIATIC AC. *(Muriaticum acidum)*
SOURCE: Hydrochloric acid
USED TO TREAT: Foot ache (page 250)

NATRUM MUR. *(Natrum muriaticum)*
SOURCE: Sodium chloride (salt)
USED TO TREAT: Anemia (page 148)

NITRIC AC. *(Nitricum acidum)*
SOURCE: Nitric acid
USED TO TREAT: Foot ache (page 250), hemorrhoids (page 299)

NUX *(Strychnos nux vomica)*
SOURCE: Poison nut tree
USED TO TREAT: Bad breath (page 182), constipation (page 221), depression (page 236), flu (page 213), heart disease (page 283), incontinence (page 324), insomnia (page 332)

PHOSPHORUS *(Phosphorus)*
SOURCE: Phosphorus
USED TO TREAT: Alzheimer's disease (page 139), anxiety (page 159), dementia (page 153), hair loss (page 268), hearing loss (page 274), periodontal disease (page 371), pneumonia (page 377)

PHOSPHORIC AC. *(Phosphoricum acidum)*
SOURCE: Phosphoric acid
USED TO TREAT: Diabetes (page 243)

PULSATILLA *(Pulsatilla nigricans)*
SOURCE: Wind flower
USED TO TREAT: Depression (page 236), flu (page 213), incontinence (page 324), menopausal symptoms (page 340), rheumatoid arthritis (page 175), varicose veins (page 392)

RHODODENDRON *(Rhododendron chrysanthum)*
SOURCE: Siberian rhododendron
USED TO TREAT: Rheumatoid arthritis (page 175)

RHUS TOX. *(Rhus toxicodendron)*
SOURCE: Poison ivy
USED TO TREAT: Heart disease (page 283), osteoarthritis (page 165)

SANGUINARIA *(Sanguinaria canadensis)*
SOURCE: Bloodroot
USED TO TREAT: Pneumonia (page 377)

SELENIUM *(Selenium)*
SOURCE: Selenium
USED TO TREAT: Hair loss (page 268)

SEPIA *(Sepia officinalis)*
SOURCE: Cuttlefish ink
USED TO TREAT: Menopausal symptoms (page 340)

SILICEA *(Silicea terra)*
SOURCE: Flint
USED TO TREAT: Cataracts (page 205), constipation (page 221), diabetes (page 243)

STAPHISAGRIA *(Delphinium staphisagria)*
SOURCE: Stavesacre
USED TO TREAT: Hysterectomy recovery (page 313)

SYMPHYTUM *(Symphytum officinale)*
SOURCE: Common comfrey
USED TO TREAT: Osteoporosis (page 358)

URTICA *(Urtica wrens)*
SOURCE: Small nettle
USED TO TREAT: Gout (page 262)

CHAPTER 5

ॐ

Acupressure:
Using Your Healing Hands

A generation ago Americans learned what the Chinese have known for more than five thousand years: Through the practice of acupressure we can use touch to stimulate the body's natural ability to heal itself.

The ancient healing arts of acupressure and acupuncture involve the use of either fingertip pressure or fine needles to activate a network of key pressure points, promoting muscle relaxation and increasing blood circulation. Healers have refined the techniques over the centuries, as they have observed and recorded the relationships between healing and touch at various points on the body.

Acupressurists and acupuncturists use two types of pressure points: local points (located where the pain occurs) and trigger points (located far from the site of the pain). Trigger points stimulate a response in distant parts of the body because they lie along a network of electrical channels (called meridians) that run throughout the body. Ancient Chinese healers have identified twelve major meridians, each named after or corresponding to a different organ, such as large intestine, small intestine, or bladder.

The meridians connect the acupressure points in what can be considered an invisible wiring system for the flow of bioelectrical impulses or the body's "essential life energy," known as *chi* or *qi* in Chinese. Traditional Chinese healers believe that chi comes in two opposite but complementary forms, yin (passive energy) and yang (active energy). When these two types of chi are balanced, the body is in harmony and in good health. When someone suffers from an injury or illness, however, chi falls out of balance. To correct an imbalance, you need to stimulate one or more of the appropriate pressure points.

Western healers may not accept the traditional explanation for how acupressure works, but the evidence shows that it does. Research shows that acupressure stimulates the release of endorphins, the body's natural painkillers and mood and immune system regulators. In fact, studies have shown that endorphin levels in the brain have doubled 30 minutes after a session of acupuncture.

Skeptics have argued that the benefits attributed to acupressure and acupuncture should be attributed instead to the placebo effect, or the ability of a patient's expectations to influence his or her experience of healing. However, studies have shown that acupuncture proves effective in pain control 55 to 85 percent of the time, much more than can be explained by the placebo effect alone.

In the hierarchy of healing, acupressure (using the fingers) ranks lowest in its ability to bring on effective healing. Acupuncture (using ultrafine needles) ranks second, and electro-acupuncture (using a mild electrical current to stimulate the acupuncture needles) stands out as most effective. In fact, studies have found that electro-acupuncture provides as much pain relief as an injection of 10 milligrams of morphine.

While not intended to replace conventional medical care, acupuncture (in the hands of a trained professional) or acupressure (as a method of self-care) can help you manage illness and control pain in many situations. As thousands of years of experience proves, when used properly, these techniques can be safe and effective in treating many illnesses.

Getting to the Point

To the beginner, acupressure can seem complex and intimidating. But once you begin to experiment with the technique, it will become very natural, and you will be able to enjoy its relaxing and healing benefits.

To help you get to the point—or more precisely, to each of the body's 365 named and numbered acupressure points—experts have developed elaborate maps of the human body, using joints, muscles, and indentations in the bones as physical landmarks. The body is symmetrical, and most acupressure points are bilateral, occurring on both sides of the body. Except when an acupressure point falls on the midline of the body, acupressure should be applied to points on both sides. (See pages 88–91 for the locations of the points.)

When practicing acupressure, you'll know you've found the correct point (also known as *tsubo*) if you feel a tingle, "charge," or electrical impulse when you apply direct pressure; the point may also feel tender. In most cases these points are located along a bone or beneath a major muscle group.

After locating the correct spot, you will use your thumbs, middle fingers, palms, or the side of your hands to apply firm, steady pressure. Your finger should be held at a right angle to the body. Start with a gentle touch and gradually push harder, until you feel a deep, even pressure but not pain. Remember that fleshy parts of the body can withstand firmer pressure than bony areas. During an acupressure session, work the points on both sides of the body to maintain balance and harmony in your body.

Three to five minutes of steady, firm pressure works best, but as little as one minute can begin to promote healing and quiet the nervous system. At the end of an acupressure session, you should feel relaxed and invigorated, but don't expect that the pain will subside or that your symptoms will disappear immediately. Acupressure isn't a matter of pressing a button and exacting a "cure"; long-term results require regular practice. It often takes at least four to six months of regular practice to see substantial pain relief for prolonged periods of time, so be patient. For the best results, plan on spending 15 minutes or so working through your acupressure points two or three times a day.

Hints for Hands-On Healing

- Before starting your acupressure session, take a few minutes to relax and get focused. If possible, settle into a quiet, warm, and well-ventilated room. Start with some deep breathing to help you relax (see page 130). During your session, try to focus your thoughts on the healing process, and visualize the pain or illness disappearing.
- If you are practicing acupressure on yourself, some points will be difficult to press without straining. To reach points on your back, place a soft tennis ball on a carpet and smoothly roll over onto it while supporting most of your weight on your elbows. If this is impossible to do without discomfort, either skip the point or recruit a friend to help.
- Keep your fingernails short to avoid scratching or poking your skin.
- Make sure to smoothly and gradually increase the pressure, and smoothly and gradually release the pressure. Avoid sharp pokes or jabs.
- Remember that acupressure should not hurt. If a

point feels painful to the touch, gradually release the pressure and move to another point.

- Avoid contact with areas that have been burned, bruised, cut, sprained, or infected. If the surrounding area is not too tender, consider applying pressure to the points near an injury to stimulate blood flow and to promote healing in the area.
- If you feel particularly stiff or tense before a session, consider soaking in a hot bath or applying a hot water bottle or heating pad to the affected area before beginning treatment.
- If possible, wait at least an hour after eating before practicing acupressure. Also avoid scheduling your acupressure sessions during times when you feel particularly hungry.

How to Find a Qualified Acupressurist or Acupuncturist

While you can practice acupressure as a self-help technique, you may want to consult a professional if you have additional questions, or if you would like to try acupuncture for a more powerful healing effect.

Nationwide, approximately three thousand medical doctors and osteopaths have studied acupuncture and use it as one of the tools in their medical practice. An additional seven thousand naturopaths and other nonphysician healers use acupressure and acupuncture. Medicaid and a number of private insurance companies cover acupuncture in some circumstances; check with your insurance company before consulting a professional to find out whether the treatment will be covered. Treatment usually costs $40 to $100 for the initial visit, and $30 to $70 for follow-up sessions; physician acupuncturists may charge more.

Acupuncture and acupressure professionals must meet state licensing or certification requirements in twenty-nine states and the District of Columbia. All states allow medical doctors to practice acupuncture, but only fourteen require physicians to have formal training in it.

If you want to use a physician acupuncturist or acupressurist, look for someone who is a member of the American Academy of Medical Acupuncture. To become a member, a physician must complete at least two hundred hours of acupuncture training and have two years' experience. Approximately three thousand doctors practice acupuncture in the United States today, but only about five hundred of them are AAMA members. For more information or a referral, contact:

American Academy of Medical Acupuncture (AAMA)
5820 Wilshire Boulevard, Suite 500
Los Angeles, CA 90036
(213) 937-5514

If you're interested in seeing a nonphysician acupuncturist or acupressurist, make sure they have been certified by the National Commission for the Certification of Acupuncturists. (A certified member can use the title Diplomate of Acupuncture, indicated by the initials *Dipl.Ac.* after his or her name.) To become certified, an acupuncturist must pass both a written and practical exam; to be eligible to take the exams, he or she must be licensed, must have at least two years of training, or must have worked as an apprentice acupuncturist for at least four years. For more information or to confirm certification of a particular acupuncturist or acupressurist, contact:

The National Commission for the Certification of Acupuncturists (NCCA)
P.O. Box 97075
Washington, DC 20090
(202) 232-1404

For additional information on acupuncture and acupressure, as well as a free referral to practitioners in your area, contact:

American Association for Acupuncture and Oriental Medicine
433 Front Street
Catasauqoa, PA 18032-2506
(610) 433-2448

Acupressure Institute of America
1533 Shattuck Avenue
Berkeley, CA 94709
(800) 442-2232
(415) 845-1059 in California

୧୬

KEY ACUPRESSURE POINTS FOR COMMON AILMENTS

BLADDER 2
USED TO TREAT: Bronchitis (page 213), colds (page 213), flu (page 213)

LOCATION: In the indentations of the eye sockets, on either side of where the bridge of the nose meets the ridge of the eyebrows

BLADDER 10
USED TO TREAT: Anxiety (page 159), arthritis (page 165), depression (page 236), osteoporosis (page 358)

LOCATION: One finger-width below the base of the skull, on the band of muscles one-half inch out from the spine.

BLADDER 15
USED TO TREAT: Heart disease (page 283)

LOCATION: Two finger-widths out on either side of the spine, level with the fifth thoracic vertebra (approximately between the shoulder blades)

BLADDER 23
USED TO TREAT: Hearing loss (page 274), impotence (page 318)

LOCATION: On the lower back, two finger-widths on either side of the spine at waist level

BLADDER 25
USED TO TREAT: Constipation (page 221)

LOCATION: Two finger-widths on either side of the spinal column, level with the top of the hipbones

BLADDER 28
USED TO TREAT: Incontinence (page 324)

LOCATION: In the lower back, two finger-widths on either side of the sacrum

BLADDER 47

USED TO TREAT: Arthritis (page 165)

LOCATION: In the lower back, between the second and third lumbar vertebrae, four finger-widths away from the spine at waist level

BLADDER 48

USED TO TREAT: Osteoporosis (page 358)

LOCATION: Two finger-widths outside the large bony area at the base of the spine, midway between the top of the hipbone and the base of the buttocks

BLADDER 60

USED TO TREAT: Foot problems (page 250)

LOCATION: In the depression behind the anklebone, on the outside edge of the ankle

BLADDER 62

USED TO TREAT: Foot problems (page 250), insomnia (page 332)

LOCATION: In the hollow directly below the outer anklebone; this point is one-third the distance from the outer anklebone to the bottom of the heel

CONCEPTION VESSEL 6

USED TO TREAT: Anxiety (page 159), constipation (page 221), impotence (page 318), incontinence (page 324), vaginal dryness (page 387)

LOCATION: Two to three finger-widths below the navel, in the middle of the abdomen

CONCEPTION VESSEL 12

USED TO TREAT: Anxiety (page 159), depression (page 236), obesity (page 352)

LOCATION: On the midline of the abdomen, halfway between the navel and the edge of the breastbone

CONCEPTION VESSEL 17

USED TO TREAT: Anxiety (page 159), heart disease (page 283), menopausal symptoms (page 340)

LOCATION: In the middle of the chest, in line with the nipples

CONCEPTION VESSEL 22

USED TO TREAT: Bronchitis (page 213), colds (page 213)

LOCATION: Just above the breastbone, in the depression below the throat

GALLBLADDER 1

USED TO TREAT: Cataracts (page 205)

LOCATION: In the slight depression level with the outside corner of the eye

GALLBLADDER 2

USED TO TREAT: Overall dental health (page 228), hearing loss (page 274), periodontal disease (page 371)

LOCATION: Behind the jawbone and in front of the earlobe, in the depression formed when the mouth is open

GALLBLADDER 8

USED TO TREAT: Hair loss (page 268)

LOCATION: Just inside the hairline, two finger-widths above the top of the ears

GALLBLADDER 12

USED TO TREAT: Insomnia (page 332)

LOCATION: Behind the ears, in the hollow under the bone

GALLBLADDER 20

USED TO TREAT: Arthritis (page 165), bronchitis (page 213), colds (page 213), hair loss (page 268)

LOCATION: Just below the base of the skull, in the hollow between the two large neck muscles, two to three inches apart, depending on the size of the head

GALLBLADDER 34

USED TO TREAT: Gallbladder disease (page 256)

LOCATION: On the outside of the leg in the hollow just beneath the meeting point of the two leg bones, one thumb-width above and two finger-widths to the outside of Stomach 36

GALLBLADDER 39

USED TO TREAT: Osteoporosis (page 358)

LOCATION: On the outside of the leg, four finger-widths above the tip of the anklebone, in the depression between the bone and the tendons

GOVERNING VESSEL 4

USED TO TREAT: Vaginal dryness (page 387)

LOCATION: On the spine between the second and third lumbar vertebrae

GOVERNING VESSEL 16

USED TO TREAT: Flu (page 213), hypertension (page 304)

LOCATION: In the center of the back of the head, in the large hollow under the base of the skull

GOVERNING VESSEL 20

USED TO TREAT: Hair loss (page 268)

LOCATION: At the top of the head, straight up from the top of the ears

GOVERNING VESSEL 26

USED TO TREAT: Depression (page 236), periodontal disease (page 371), vaginal dryness (page 387)

LOCATION: Halfway up the groove below the nose

HEART 3

USED TO TREAT: Heart disease (page 283)

LOCATION: On the inside of the elbow, at the inside edge of the crease when the elbow is flexed

HEART 7

USED TO TREAT: Anxiety (page 159), heart disease (page 283), insomnia (page 332)

LOCATION: With your palms facing upward, on the little-finger side of the forearm, in the hollow at the crease of the wrist

KIDNEY 1

USED TO TREAT: Foot problems (page 250), hypertension (page 304), impotence (page 318), menopausal symptoms (page 340)

LOCATION: On the sole of the foot, in the depression just below the ball of the foot

KIDNEY 3

USED TO TREAT: Hair loss (page 268), impotence (page 318), incontinence (page 324), toothache (page 228)

LOCATION: Inside the ankle, in the depression halfway between the anklebone and the back of the ankle

KIDNEY 6

USED TO TREAT: Insomnia (page 332), varicose veins (page 392)

LOCATION: Directly below the inside of the anklebone, in a slight indentation

LARGE INTESTINE 4

USED TO TREAT: Arthritis (page 165), constipation (page 221), flu (page 213), hemorrhoids (page 299), menopausal symptoms (page 340), toothache (page 228)

LOCATION: On the outside of the hand, in the webbing between the thumb and index finger, at the highest spot of the muscle when the thumb and index finger are brought closest together

LARGE INTESTINE 11

USED TO TREAT: Arthritis (page 165), constipation (page 221), hemorrhoids (page 299)

LOCATION: At the outer edge of the elbow crease; in the

depression at the end of the elbow crease, when the elbow is slightly bent

Liver 3

USED TO TREAT: Depression (page 236), hypertension (page 304)

LOCATION: On the top of the foot, in the web between the first and second toe

Lung 5

USED TO TREAT: Bronchitis (page 213), colds (page 213)

LOCATION: On the inside of the elbow, in the hollow on the outer edge of the tendons when the elbow is slightly bent

Lung 9

USED TO TREAT: Arthritis (page 165), pneumonia (page 377)

LOCATION: In the hollow on the inside wrist crease, just below the base of the thumb

Lung 10

USED TO TREAT: Arthritis (page 165)

LOCATION: On the palm side of the hand, in the center of the pad at the base of the thumb

Pericardium 4

USED TO TREAT: Heart disease (page 283)

LOCATION: On the inside of the forearm, halfway between the wrist and the elbow, in line with the middle finger, in the depression between the tendons

Pericardium 6

USED TO TREAT: Anxiety (page 159), heart disease (page 283)

LOCATION: In the middle of the inside of the forearm, between the tendons, three finger-widths up from the wrist case

PERICARDIUM 7

USED TO TREAT: Arthritis (page 165)

LOCATION: In the middle of the inside wrist crease

SMALL INTESTINE 19

USED TO TREAT: Hearing loss (page 274), toothache (page 228)

LOCATION: In the depression directly in front of the ear opening; the depression becomes deeper when the mouth is opened

SPLEEN 4

USED TO TREAT: Obesity (page 352)

LOCATION: On the arch of the foot, one thumb-width from the ball of the foot toward the heel

SPLEEN 6

USED TO TREAT: Incontinence (page 324), menopausal symptoms (page 340), varicose veins (page 392)

LOCATION: On the inside of the leg, four finger-widths above the tip of the anklebone and just inside the bone of the leg

SPLEEN 8

USED TO TREAT: Constipation (page 221)

LOCATION: On the inside of the lower leg, four finger-widths below the knee, in the depression under the bone

SPLEEN 9

USED TO TREAT: Varicose veins (page 392)

LOCATION: On the inside of the leg, below the knee and under the large bulge of bone

SPLEEN 10

USED TO TREAT: Varicose veins (page 392)

LOCATION: On the inside edge of the top of the knee, where the opposite thumb touches the muscles when the knee is flexed

Spleen 12

USED TO TREAT: Impotence (page 318)

LOCATION: In the center of the crease where the leg joins the trunk

Spleen 16

USED TO TREAT: Obesity (page 352)

LOCATION: On the lower edge of the rib cage, one-half inch in from the nipple line

Stomach 1

USED TO TREAT: Cataracts (page 205)

LOCATION: Directly below the pupil of the eye, in the center of the ridge of the bony socket below the eye

Stomach 3

USED TO TREAT: Bronchitis (page 213), colds (page 213), overall dental health (page 228), periodontal disease (page 371)

LOCATION: At the bottom of the cheekbone, directly below the pupil and level with the outside edge of the nostril

Stomach 4

USED TO TREAT: Overall dental health (page 228)

LOCATION: Just below Stomach 3, at the corner of the mouth

Stomach 6

USED TO TREAT: Periodontal disease (page 371)

LOCATION: Along the lower angle of the jawbone, in the depression formed by the muscles and tendons when the teeth are clenched

Stomach 7

USED TO TREAT: Toothache (page 228)

LOCATION: On the side of the cheek, in the hollow along the cheekbone and in front of the earlobe

Stomach 8

USED TO TREAT: Cataracts (page 205)

LOCATION: At the corner of the forehead, one finger-width inside the hairline

Stomach 34
USED TO TREAT: Constipation (page 221)
LOCATION: Three finger-widths above the kneecap, in the depression on the outer edge of the muscle

Stomach 36
USED TO TREAT: Arthritis (page 165), heart disease (page 283), hemorrhoids (page 299)
LOCATION: Four finger-widths below the kneecap and one finger-width outside the shinbone

Triple Warmer 4
USED TO TREAT: Arthritis (page 165)
LOCATION: In the hollow in the center of the wrist case, on the outside of the arm

Triple Warmer 5
USED TO TREAT: Arthritis (page 165), hearing loss (page 274), menopausal symptoms (page 340)
LOCATION: On the outside of the forearm, two finger-widths down from the wrist crease, between the forearm bones

Triple Warmer 15
USED TO TREAT: Arthritis (page 165), bronchitis (page 213), colds (page 213), flu (page 213)
LOCATION: Midway between the base of the neck and the outside of the shoulders, one-half inch below the top of the shoulders

Triple Warmer 21
USED TO TREAT: Hearing loss (page 274), overall dental health (page 228)
LOCATION: In the depression in front of the notch at the top of the ear; the depression will deepen when the mouth is opened

TRIPLE WARMER 23

USED TO TREAT: Cataracts (page 205)

LOCATION: In the slight depression at the outer edge of the eyebrow

KEY
B—Bladder
CV—Conception Vessel
GB—Gallbladder
GV—Governing Vessel
H—Heart
K—Kidney
LI—Large Intestine
L—Liver
Lu—Lung
P—Pericardium
SI—Small Intestine
Sp—Spleen
St—Stomach
TW—Triple Warmer

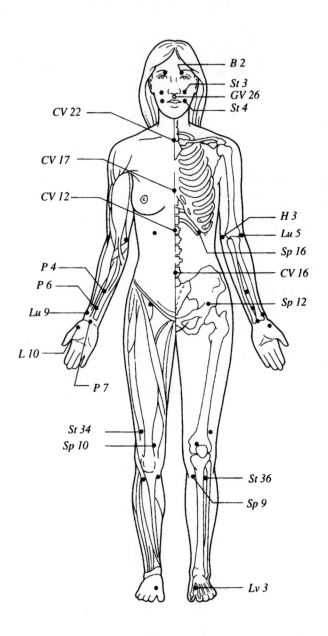

B 2

St 3
GV 26
St 4

CV 22

CV 17

CV 12

H 3
Lu 5
Sp 16

P 4
P 6
Lu 9
L 10
P 7

CV 16

Sp 12

St 34
Sp 10

St 36
Sp 9

Lv 3

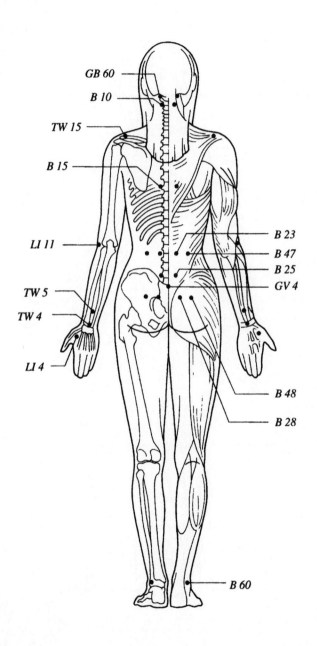

GB 60

B 10

TW 15

B 15

LI 11

TW 5

TW 4

LI 4

B 23

B 47

B 25

GV 4

B 48

B 28

B 60

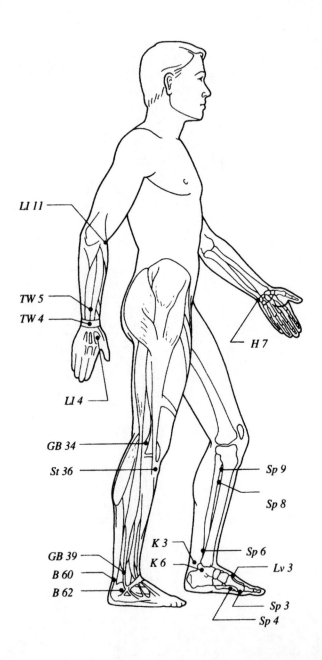

LI 11

TW 5

TW 4

H 7

LI 4

GB 34

St 36

Sp 9

Sp 8

K 3

GB 39

K 6

Sp 6

Lv 3

B 60

B 62

Sp 3

Sp 4

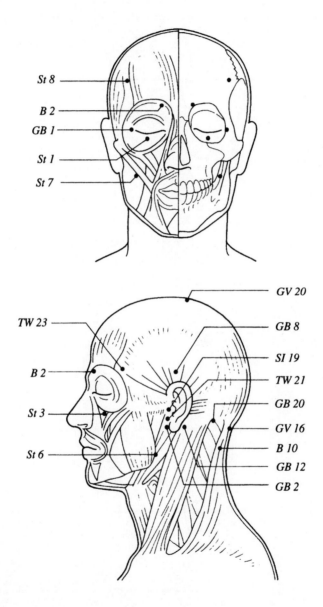

PART TWO

GRAYING GRACEFULLY

PART TWO

READING GRATEFULLY

CHAPTER 6

Using Your Body: Exercise for Lifelong Fitness

Growing older is hard on your body. Unless you take steps to preserve your physical fitness, over the years you will lose muscle mass and bone density while gaining body fat and excess pounds. You will experience a decline in aerobic capacity, a decline in muscle strength, and a decline in flexibility. Fortunately there is an easy way to stop the clock: exercise.

Exercise offers some of the best protection against many of the infirmities and illnesses associated with aging. Many experts even suggest that some chronic complaints once thought to be major health problems may in fact be simply symptoms of disuse.

You undoubtedly know you should exercise, but you may not fully appreciate how important exercise can be to your overall health. No matter what your age, exercise can improve your physical and emotional health, reduce your risk of serious illness, and make you look years younger than your chronological age. Studies have shown that moderate exercise strengthens the body's defenses against disease; after a workout the number and aggressiveness of the white blood cells increase by 50 to 300 percent. In addition, exercise can:

- reduce your risk of developing certain cancers, cardio-vascular disease, colds and upper respiratory tract infections, diabetes (noninsulin dependent), high blood pressure, obesity, osteoarthritis, osteoporosis, and stroke;
- relieve anxiety, constipation, depression, low-back pain, and stress; and
- improve your cholesterol levels; flexibility; immune system; mental alertness and reaction time; mood; muscle strength; self-esteem; sexual desire, performance, and satisfaction; short-term memory; sleep; state of relaxation; vision; and overall quality of life.

You don't have to spend hours in the gym to enjoy these benefits of exercise. Recent studies have shown that as little as 30 minutes a day of light physical activity will reduce your risk of disease by lowering blood pressure and cholesterol. Yes, that's physical activity, not hard-core exercise. The time you spend strolling the neighborhood, walking the dog, climbing the stairs, and mowing the lawn counts toward your goal. Other studies have shown that you don't even have to do your 30 minutes of activity all at once, as long as you total a half hour during the course of the day.

Of course, these studies looked at minimum levels of exercise. To enjoy all the benefits of exercise, you'll have to work harder and longer. But the point is that with even a nominal level of exertion, you can enjoy major life-saving improvements in your overall health.

Designing a Workout

A well-rounded exercise program strives to build aerobic fitness, muscle strength, and flexibility. While you won't necessarily do all types of exercise during every workout, your weekly routine should include all three types of exercise.

Aerobic Fitness

If you don't exercise regularly, you have almost certainly lost aerobic power—and you probably know it. Without exercise you will steadily lose aerobic conditioning throughout your thirties, forties, and fifties. By age 65 the average person's aerobic capacity has dropped by about 40 percent, compared to the relatively fit days of young adulthood. Climbing a flight of stairs or walking through an airport concourse—activity that once caused little exertion—might now leave you winded and strained.

The term *aerobic* means "using oxygen." During aerobic exercise your heart and lungs work harder than normal to provide your muscles with the oxygen they demand, and you must breathe heavily and steadily to meet your body's increased need for oxygen. During anaerobic exercise your heart and lungs cannot meet your body's oxygen demands for longer than a short burst of activity, and you are left gasping and wheezing for breath (even if you're in good shape). Jogging around a track is aerobic exercise; sprinting to catch the bus is anaerobic exercise. No one—not even Carl Lewis—can do anaerobic exercise for more than a couple of minutes.

To improve your level of aerobic fitness and strengthen your heart and lungs, you need to perform some type of aerobic exercise, such as walking, jogging, bicycling, swimming, cross-country skiing, aerobic dancing, or rope skipping. These activities involve the rhythmic, repeated use of the major muscle groups. When done regularly—three times a week for at least 20 to 30 minutes—aerobic activities improve the efficiency of the heart, lungs, and muscles and increase their ability to do work and withstand stress.

Regular aerobic exercise helps lower your pulse rate, both during exercise and at rest. As your heart grows larger and stronger, it pumps more blood with each beat, decreasing blood pressure. One study found that older people who had already suffered a heart attack reduced their risk of a second attack by 20 to 25 percent when they started to exercise. These heart-saving benefits show up after as little as six to ten weeks of regular aerobic exercise.

For maximum benefit you need to work hard enough— but not too hard. Your pulse rate, or the number of heart-beats per minute, is your body's speedometer: It tells you how fast your heart is going and if you need to speed up or slow things down to exercise in your optimal conditioning zone. Cardiovascular conditioning takes place when your heart beats at 70 to 85 percent of its maximum safe rate. Your maximum heart rate is approximately 220 minus your age. (See table on pages 98–99.) You should take your pulse before starting to exercise, again after exercising for 10 or 15 minutes, and immediately after stopping.

Measure your heart rate at any place where you can feel your pulse. Two easy pulse points are the inside wrist and the carotid artery in the neck. Using a stopwatch, count your pulse for 10 seconds, then multiply that number by six to get the number of beats per minute. During exercise a pulse that is under your target range indicates you should speed up or work harder, while one that is higher means you should slow down. Another simple test: You should be able to talk comfortably during exercise; if you can't carry on a conversation, you're working too hard.

TARGET PULSE RANGES

AGE	MAXIMUM HEART RATE	TARGET RANGE
40	180	126–153
45	175	122–140

50	170	119–145
55	165	115–140
60	160	112–136
65	155	109–132
70	150	105–128
75	145	102–123
80	140	98–119
85	135	95–115
90	130	91–110

If you're new to exercise, start slow. Try 10 minutes of light to moderate exercise three times a week and gradually extend your workout time to 20 or 30 minutes, then increase the intensity. Consider a low-impact activity; as we get older, the shock-absorbing fat pads in the feet thin out and the cushioning disks in the spine dry up, making high-intensity exercise more punishing on the joints.

Aim for workouts of moderate intensity—about 70 percent of your maximum heart rate. If you work at the higher end of the exercise benefit zone, you will experience a faster improvement in your athletic ability, but this extra effort won't markedly improve your health, and it greatly increases your risk of injury. The death rates from cardiovascular disease, cancer, and diabetes are much lower in moderate exercisers than in nonexercisers, but only slightly lower in heavy exercisers. In addition, moderate exercise reduces stress, anxiety, and blood pressure as effectively as strenuous exercise does.

Be sure to warm up for 5 to 10 minutes by doing light calisthenics before your aerobic workout. You might also go through the motions of the main workout at a slower pace as a warm-up.

Also remember to cool down. After your workout walk

slowly for 3 to 5 minutes, or until your heart rate returns to just 10 or 15 beats above the resting rate. (The less fit you are, the more time you'll need for a cool-down.) Stopping suddenly can cause the blood to pool in the legs, reducing blood pressure and possibly causing fainting or even a heart attack.

Muscle Strength

Many people assume that muscles atrophy over the years, but this doesn't have to be the case. You can keep your muscles strong and supple by performing strength-building exercises, such as weight lifting and isometric exercises.

Without strength training, you will lose muscle mass and strength: The average American loses 10 to 20 percent of muscle strength between the ages of 20 and 50, and then another 25 to 30 percent between 50 and 70. In addition, every decade from age 40 on, the average person loses six pounds of muscle; this change in body composition from muscle to fat can change the shape of your body even if it doesn't change your weight on the scales, because muscle is denser than fat.

Strength training helps stave off changes in body composition by raising the basal metabolic rate, or the number of calories the body burns at rest. The more muscle you have, the higher your metabolic rate, the more calories you burn, and the easier it is to fight flab. At age 20 the average woman has 23 percent body fat; the average man, 18 percent. At 35, those fat figures have jumped to 30 percent and 25 percent, respectively. And by age 60, the average woman is 44 percent fat and the average man is 38 percent fat. That increase in fat corresponds to a decrease in muscle mass over the years.

To slow this shift from muscle to fat, you must do strength-building exercises, not just aerobic exercise. Studies have shown that people who maintain their aerobic fitness still lose muscle mass—about one pound of muscle every two years after age 20—if they don't diversify their workouts to include strength training.

In addition to keeping you lean, strength training has other benefits:

- It makes it easier to perform simple tasks such as carrying groceries, opening jars, and climbing stairs.
- It decreases the risk of falls and injury.
- It strengthens the joints.
- It helps build bone mass and fights osteoporosis.

In fact, regular strength training can virtually stop the aging process when it comes to muscles. For example, one study found that 70-year-old men who had been strength-training since middle age were just as strong, on average, as 28-year-old men who didn't strength-train.

You're never too old to grow stronger. And the more out of shape you are, the greater your proportional gain will be. Frail octogenarians can easily double or triple their strength in just a couple of months. One study found that 90-year-old nursing home residents increased their muscle strength by up to 180 percent in an eight-week exercise program.

High-resistance exercise offers impressive benefits, even at age 101. When done properly, weight training has no great risk of injury or pain. And you can build as much—or more—muscle than you had in your twenties.

Training Tips

- Your training weight should be 70 to 80 percent of the maximum weight that you can lift. So if the heaviest weight you can lift in a certain maneuver is 50 pounds, your training weight for that exercise would be 35 to 40 pounds. You should be able to lift that weight eight to twelve times. Once you can lift a weight twenty times, it's time to move up to a heavier weight.
- One set of each exercise is almost as effective as multiple sets in building muscle and boosting metabolism. However, to build muscle faster, follow a high-intensity strategy: After finishing the set, reduce the weight by 10 pounds and perform as many extra repetitions as you can (usually three

or four). One two-month study found that people who followed the high-intensity strategy were able to lift 25 pounds more than before, compared to a 15-pound improvement among those who followed the one-set approach.

- Three workouts per week is the basic recommendation for building muscle; however, you should be able to maintain your current level of strength with two strength-training sessions a week.

- To make muscles grow, work to the point of muscle failure. Some experts believe the body needs to build up lactic acids inside the muscle cells to stimulate growth. Others believe that heavy weights tear the muscle apart and cause it to form new muscle fibers.

- Take it slow and easy. Each repetition of an exercise should take about 6 seconds—2 seconds for the first half of the maneuver and 4 for the return to the original position.

- Use good form. Doing an exercise incorrectly can cause muscle damage and injury.

- Don't hold your breath. Holding your breath can cause a dangerous rise in blood pressure, then a sudden drop when you release your breath, possibly causing lightheadedness or fainting. Inhale, then exhale during the exertion phase of the movement, and inhale during the release.

- Be wary of free weights. Start with weight-lifting machines or elastic exercise bands if your strength or balance has declined, since free weights can be dangerous if dropped.

Flexibility

Flexibility is a critical part of fitness but one that is often overlooked. Flexibility involves more than touching your toes; it involves maintaining the range of motion in your joints, which can allow you to perform your everyday activities without discomfort. It also makes you less prone to muscle strains, sprains, and tears. The only way to preserve your flexibility is to perform stretching exercises regularly.

Without regular stretching, the average adult's flexibility declines by 5 percent per decade. Over the years that steady loss in flexibility can make it difficult to stoop over to pick up something dropped on the floor or to look behind you when driving.

As little as 10 minutes of stretching every other day can help to prevent stiffness and loss of flexibility. Don't stretch "cold" muscles. Instead, stretch 2 or 3 minutes into your warm-up, just after you have broken a sweat. Stretch for 2 minutes before aerobic activities and 10 minutes before abrupt stop-and-go activities, such as tennis or basketball. You don't need to stretch before strength training, but you should afterward. Regardless of the type of exercise you perform, after your workout stretch 2 minutes for every 10 minutes of your workout time.

To build flexibility, bend or flex until you feel tension or slight discomfort—but not pain—and hold each stretch for 20 to 60 seconds. Do not hold your breath, and do not bounce or pulse, which can tear the connective tissue in the joints.

Building strength and increasing flexibility are not mutually exclusive. This myth has been perpetuated by people who build muscle and fail to work at stretching.

Getting Started

No matter what your age, it's never too late to start exercising, but don't expect to overcome decades of inactivity in a couple of weeks. It took a long time to get out of shape, and it will take some time to get back in shape, so be patient with yourself. You'll start to feel the physical and emotional benefits of exercise in a few weeks, and your fitness level will continue to improve over the next few months. Studies have shown that a year of regular exercise can return the body to a fitness level of ten years earlier.

To get into shape, you will have to make a commitment to exercise regularly; sporadic exercise won't bring the rewards of fitness. Your body will adapt to the physical demands you place on it, and it will do so without injury or discomfort, if you exercise sensibly. If you're not used to lifting anything heavier than a 10-pound bag of groceries, you'll find it difficult to lift a 20-pound barbell. But if you push yourself gradually, your body will adjust: Your muscles will become stronger, and your heart and lungs will begin to work more efficiently.

You can push yourself and overload your muscles in one of three ways: by increasing the intensity of exercise (the amount of weight you lift or the speed you run), the duration of exercise (the length of time you work out), or the frequency of exercise (the number of workouts per week). As a rule of thumb, limit your overload to no more than 10 percent per week to allow your body to adjust to your fitness program gradually.

You need to space your workouts for maximum benefits. If you perform aerobic exercise fewer than three times a week, you will not achieve adequate aerobic conditioning. However, if you work out five times or more, you run a much higher risk of injury and only a nominal additional increase in fitness. Perform your aerobic exercise every other day, with the strength-training sessions in between.

If you have coronary disease or take medications regularly, consult your doctor before starting an exercise program. Also talk to your doctor if you're a smoker, if you haven't had a checkup in more than two years, if you're more than 20 pounds overweight, or if you have a risk factor for coronary disease, such as diabetes, lung disease, hypertension, high levels of LDL cholesterol or low levels of HDL cholesterol, or a family history of early heart attack.

Once you start exercising, keep at it. Consistency counts. If you miss a few days of exercise, don't feel guilty and throw in the towel (literally). Instead, just get back to it, but don't try to make up for lost time by increasing the intensity of your workout. In fact, if you skip exercise for one week, cut back on the intensity of your workout and gradually build up again. You start to lose aerobic conditioning and strength if you sit it out for as little as one week.

Bottoms Up

Don't rely on your thirst to tell you when to drink during exercise: The older you get, the less reliable your thirst detector becomes. Instead, drink two 8-ounce cups of water about two hours before exercise, another cup every 20 minutes during exercise, and an additional cup or two within a half hour after your workout.

In the body water helps to regulate body temperature, carry nutrients, remove toxins and waste materials, maintain blood volume, and facilitate chemical reactions in the cells. If you're a couch potato, your body loses 64 to 80 ounces—eight to ten 8-ounce glasses—of water a day. This fluid loss comes from urination, defecation, perspiration, and even respiration. (The body loses water vapor each time you exhale.) If you exercise, you lose even more, depending on the intensity and duration of your workout, as well as the weather and conditions where you're exercising.

To replace this water loss, make a point to drink eight to ten 8-ounce glasses of water per day, in addition to the extra fluids consumed during exercise. One simple way to tell whether you're drinking enough is to check the color and quantity of your urine. If it's dark and scant, you're not drinking enough and your body has to concentrate waste products in a relatively small quantity of water. As a rule, you should pass pale yellow urine about four times a day.

CHAPTER 7

❧

Fueling Your Body:
Nutrition for Optimal Health

Food is not only fuel for the body but medicine as well. Eating the right foods provides energy for the day's activities and also protects against a number of illnesses often associated with aging, including heart disease, cancer, arthritis, osteoporosis, cataracts, and others.

There is no single food prescription that works for everyone. The key, of course, is balance. We all have different nutritional needs and food preferences, and the challenge is to structure a diet plan that includes both the foods we should eat and the foods we want to eat.

Four types of nutrients—carbohydrates, proteins, fats, and vitamins and minerals—work together to nourish our bodies and provide the raw materials necessary for all our bodily processes. (Vitamins and minerals are discussed in detail in Chapter 3.)

Carbohydrates are the body's major source of energy. There are two types: simple carbohydrates (sugars), which are quickly converted to blood sugar, and complex carbo-hydrates (starches), which are metabolized more slowly and provide a more gradual supply of energy. Generally speaking, about half of the calories you consume each day should be carbohydrates, especially complex carbohy-drates, such as whole-grain breads, legumes, cereals, pasta, potatoes, and other vegetables. When it comes to eating simple carbohydrates, try to stick to fruits, which offer vita-mins and minerals in addition to sugar, rather than refined sugar, honey, and corn syrup. Remember that sugar is sugar, whether it goes by the name sucrose, fructose, or maltose—and one is not better or worse for you than an-other.

Proteins consist of chains of amino acids, which the body uses to perform metabolic functions and to build and main-tain body tissues. The older we get, the less protein we need, but the less efficient our bodies become at extracting it from the foods we eat. As a result, rather than eating less protein, we need to eat more as we age, starting at around age 50. Strive to eat about 12 percent of your total calories from protein. Complete proteins (those with complete amino acids) are found in animal and plant products such as meats, fish, poultry, and dairy products. Other foods—such as legumes, grains, nuts, and seeds—are also good sources of protein.

Fats, though often vilified, are essential to human health. They are needed for growth, hormone production, and other essential body processes. They also carry and store fat-soluble vitamins (vitamins A, D, E, and K). And, of course, fats make food more palatable by adding flavor, aroma, and texture. When consumed in excess, fats also contribute to a number of health problems.

All Fats Are Not Created Equal

Experts estimate that high-fat diets contribute to at least 300,000 deaths a year. Dietary fat has been linked to ath-erosclerosis and heart disease, elevated blood cholesterol, high blood pressure, diabetes, arthritis, multiple sclerosis, several types of cancer, and of course, obesity.

The typical American consumes about 40 percent of calories from fat, despite warnings that fat intake should be limited to 30 percent of calories or lower. That means about 60 to 80 grams of fat for a 1,800- to 2,400-calorie daily diet. (One gram of fat has 9 calories; one gram of protein or carbohydrate has four calories.) But for people at risk of heart disease, a diet consisting of 30 percent fat may be too much. The body needs only about 10 percent of calories from fat (about 20 grams a day) to perform its necessary functions.

In addition to watching total fat, you must also keep an eye out for the type of fat you are consuming. Dietary fats consist of combinations of three types of fatty acids—saturated, polyunsaturated, and monounsaturated:

- **Saturated fats** tend to be hard at room temperature.
  Examples: Butter, cheese, chocolate, coconut oil, egg yolk, lard, meat, palm oil, vegetable shortening
- **Polyunsaturated fats** tend to be liquid at room temperature.
  Examples: Corn, cottonseed, fish, safflower, soybean, sunflower oils
- **Monounsaturated fats** fall in between.
  Examples: Avocado, canola, cashew, olive, and peanut oils

Saturated fats should be avoided as much as possible. These fats raise the level of cholesterol in the blood, which increases the risk of heart disease. In addition, saturated fats (which usually come from animals) tend to contain large amounts of cholesterol. You should worry less about differentiating between mono- and polyunsaturated fats and instead focus your attention on limiting your overall fat intake, paying special care to cut out saturated fats.

Also beware of trans fatty acids, which are formed when liquid oils are converted to solid fat to make margarine and vegetable shortening. In an attempt to respond to health concerns about saturated fats, food manufacturers have created trans fats by bubbling hydrogen through vegetable oil in a process known as hydrogenation. The resulting partially hydrogenated vegetable oils form a semisolid spread (like margarine), but they contain minimal amounts of saturated fat. While billed as a heart-smart alternative to butter since it contains little saturated fat and no cholesterol (since it came from a vegetable rather than an animal), research shows that these trans fats may be as hazardous to your health and heart as old-fashioned saturated fats. One study has found that cooking with margarine (instead of liquid oil) increases the risk of heart disease by nearly 90 percent. Other studies have found that women who eat high levels of trans fatty acids are at greater risk of developing breast cancer and that men who eat them are more susceptible to prostate cancer.

This raises the butter-versus-margarine question: Which is better (or less bad) for you, butter (a saturated fat) or margarine (a trans fat)? Well, it depends.

- If you're concerned about your cholesterol level, choose margarine (which is made from vegetable oil and does not contain cholesterol). Choose a soft, tub-style margarine, since these products are less hydrogenated and contain fewer trans fatty acids than stick margarines do. (Unfortunately, manufacturers don't list trans fats on nutrition labels, so you can't compare products.)
- If you're concerned about saturated fat but need a stick product, choose stick margarine. Margarine tends to be lower in saturated fat than butter; for example, 1 tablespoon of stick butter contains about 7 grams of saturated fat, compared with about 2 grams in 1 tablespoon of stick margarine.
- If you can't live without the taste of butter, go for the real thing, but consider using a whipped product. Because of all the added air, 1 tablespoon of whipped butter contains about 4 grams of saturated fat, compared with 7 grams in a stick product.

- If you're counting calories, choose a diet margarine or spread. They contain more water and less fat per tablespoon. (Because of the high water content, they aren't a good alternative when cooking.)

Don't assume that Olestra, the so-called "fake fat," offers a realistic alternative. Olestra has been test-marketed in several types of snack foods, including Fat-Free Pringles and Frito-Lay's Max Chips. (To identify a food containing Olestra, look for the Olean logo on the front of the package.) Olestra looks, tastes, and acts like real fat, but the human digestive system cannot break it down, so it passes through the body without being absorbed or adding to the tally of total calories for the day. However, Olestra does not make its way through the body unnoticed. During its journey through the digestive system, it steals from the body the fat-soluble vitamins A, D, E, and K, as well as carotenoids, important antioxidants.

You don't have to overindulge to suffer from Olestra's negative side effects. One study found that as few as six Olestra prepared potato chips (about 3 grams) caused a 20 percent drop in levels of beta-carotene and a 38 percent drop in lycopene, another carotenoid. It can also create most unpleasant side effects, including anal leakage, diarrhea, intestinal cramping, and flatulence.

The bottom line: Don't look for dietary shortcuts. To protect your health and avoid a number of illnesses, limit your fat intake to no more than 30 percent of calories from fat, with no more than 10 percent from saturated fats.

A Word About Fiber

While not a nutrient, dietary fiber is a necessary part of a well-balanced diet. Studies show that people who eat high-fiber diets have a lower risk of developing heart disease, high cholesterol, obesity, certain cancers, gallbladder disease, diverticulosis, and chronic disease of the colon.

Dietary fiber consists of complex carbohydrates and natural polymers (such as lignin), which give structure and shape to plants. There are two types of fiber—soluble and insoluble—both of which are found in fruits, vegetables, legumes, and whole grains.

Soluble fiber dissolves in the digestive tract, forming a gellike material that helps lower cholesterol levels and that traps carcinogens and eliminates them from the body. Foods high in soluble fiber include oats, kidney beans, citrus fruits, apples, and potatoes.

Insoluble fiber, as the name implies, does not break down as it moves through the digestive system. This type of fiber provides the stools with the soft bulk required to absorb body waste; it also helps the intestines work smoothly and speeds the movement of the stools through the intestines. Insoluble fiber becomes increasingly important as we grow older, because the intestines lose elasticity, increasing the tendency toward constipation. Wheat bran and whole grains, as well as the skins of many fruits and vegetables, are rich sources of this type of fiber.

Current guidelines recommend that the average adult consume at least 25 grams of fiber daily by eating a diet rich in fruits, vegetables, and whole grains. A 1996 study published in *The Journal of the American Medical Association* found that men who ate more than 25 grams of fiber per day had a 36 percent lower risk of developing heart disease than those who consumed less than 15 grams. The study found that every 10 grams of fiber added to the diet lowered the risk of heart attack by 19 percent.

Increase your dietary fiber a little at a time, over a period of several weeks. Too much fiber at once can cause intestinal bloating, gas, and cramps in some people. Be sure to increase your fluid intake when you increase fiber, to keep your stools soft and to avoid constipation. In general, the less processed or refined a food is, the more fiber it contains.

You can boost your fiber intake by eating the skins of potatoes, apples, and other fruits and vegetables with edible skins (after washing them thoroughly, of course). Also opt for brown rice instead of white and whole-wheat flour instead of white. When cooking, stir-fry or steam vegetables to minimize breakdown of fiber. And add wheat germ to hot or cold cereals, sprinkle it in yogurt, mix it into casseroles, or substitute it for up to a half-cup of the flour in most baked goods.

The Healing Power of Phytochemicals

Your mother was right: Eating fruits, vegetables, and grains is good for you. Study after study has shown that people who eat plenty of plant foods tend to suffer less from cardiovascular disease, cancer, and many other illnesses, compared with people who eat lots of meat and dairy products. Of course, plant foods tend to be high in vitamins, minerals, and fiber and low in fat and calories, but there seems to be more to it than that. Researchers now suspect they know what gives plant foods their added healing power: phytochemicals, or plant chemicals.

There are hundreds of different phytochemicals, only a small number of which have been studied. To the best of our understanding, they work as part of a plant's antioxidant defense system, and they also help the plant survive viral attack and difficult weather. In humans phytochemicals have no known nutritional value, and they do not add to the caloric content of food. But they do seem to have a remarkable ability to help fight disease.

Phytochemicals include flavonoids, chlorophylline, dithiolthiones, indoles, isoflavones, isothiocyanates, lignans, saponins, sulfur compounds, and other substances with polysyllabic names. While each of these chemicals performs a very specific task, as a group they are marvelous at fighting cancer by preventing cell damage and by suppressing malignant changes in the cells when they do occur.

All plants contain a number of phytochemicals. While some phytochemicals have been isolated and offered for sale as nutrition supplements, it is best to get your daily dose of phytochemicals by eating a diet high in fruits and vegetables. At this point scientists do not know whether specific phytochemicals act alone to fight disease, or whether they work synergistically with other plant chemicals. So listen to your mother and eat your vegetables.

From the Pantry to the Plate

You may assume that eating right means simply choosing the "right" foods, but the choices you make when buying, storing, and preparing food can go a long way toward enhancing—or undermining—its nutritional value. Consider the following tips:

- The whole is greater . . . When shopping for cereals and grains, avoid products made with white flour; instead, choose foods made of whole grains. During the milling process, grains lose most of their vitamins and minerals, though some are added to "enriched" products.
- Fresh or frozen? In an ideal world, your fruits and vegetables would arrive on your plate just hours after leaving the field or garden. But in the real world, produce spends days or weeks in transit, losing vitamins and minerals each day. If you're in doubt about the freshness of the produce in your market, don't hesitate to choose frozen. The flash-freezing process used to prepare frozen foods protects all the vitamins except vitamin E. Look for products frozen in plastic cooking pouches.
- Can the canned vegetables. Water-soluble vitamins leach out of the vegetables and into the water that canned vegetables are packed in, robbing them of their nutritional value. Avoid canned vegetables and fruits except when absolutely necessary. For the same reason, avoid soaking vegetables for extended periods before cooking, and steam rather than boil them to preserve their vitamin content.
- Reduce, reuse, recycle. If you prepare produce by boiling, use as little water as possible and reuse the

water for gravies, sauces, and stocks, since this water contains many of the vitamins (as well as the flavors) of the foods cooked in it. In the morning you might also consider drinking the milk at the bottom of the cereal bowl, since this runoff contains many of the vitamins added to fortified cereals.

- You can never be too rich, too thin, or too cold. Set the temperature in your freezer at 0 degrees F or less. At higher temperatures, foods begin to thaw, and then they lose some of their vitamins.

- Don't let the sun shine. To protect the riboflavin content, store milk and bread away from strong light. Avoid milk in clear glass bottles for this reason.

- Less really is more. No matter what you're cooking, use the minimum cooking time necessary. To preserve vitamin content, high temperatures over a short period of time beats low temperatures over a longer period of time.

- Bigger is better. Vegetables lose less vitamin content if they are cooked whole rather than in pieces. To preserve vitamin content, cook first, then cut.

The Mysteries of the Pyramid

As the federal government's food pyramid reminds us, grains, fruits, and vegetables should be the cornerstone of a healthy diet. The Food Guide Pyramid, published by the Department of Agriculture in 1992, offers guidance for what healthy Americans two years of age and older should eat.

The pyramid is divided into a number of food groups, each with a suggested number of servings. However, within the groups some foods are better choices than others, as this table shows:

FATS, OILS, AND SWEETS: USE SPARINGLY

Best choices
   Nonfat spreads
Acceptable choices
   Light margarine; olive, canola, and vegetable oils; fruit-snack candies, hard candies, honey, molasses, sorbet, syrups; low-fat cookies, cakes, and pies

Less preferable choices
Butter, lard, stick margarine; coconut, palm, and other tropical oils; candy bars, chocolate, cakes, cookies, and pies

DAIRY: 2 TO 3 SERVINGS PER DAY
(A serving is approximately 1 cup of liquid milk or yogurt, or 1 to 1½ ounces of cheese.)
Best choices
Skim or 1% milk, buttermilk, or cottage cheese; nonfat yogurt; nonfat cheese; nonfat dairy desserts
Acceptable choices
2% milk, buttermilk, or cottage cheese; low-fat yogurt, cheese, dairy desserts
Less preferable choices
Whole milk, 4% fat cottage cheese; regular cheese, regular frozen desserts

MEAT: 2 TO 3 SERVINGS
(A serving is 2 to 3 ounces of cooked lean meat, 3 to 4 ounces of tofu, 2 large eggs, 1 cup cooked beans, or 4 tablespoons of peanut butter.)
Best choices
Extralean meats; pork tenderloin; skinless chicken breast; turkey breast, drumstick, or skinless wing; shellfish; lean fish; nonfat hot dogs or lunch meats
Acceptable choices
Lean meats; skinless chicken drumstick; turkey with skin or thigh without skin; low-fat hot dogs or lunch meats
Less preferable choices
Beef brisket, rib roast, regular ground beef; spareribs, ground pork sausage; chicken with skin; chicken liver; ground turkey; duck; goose; regular hot dogs or lunch meats

VEGETABLES: 3 TO 5 SERVINGS PER DAY
(A serving is ½ cup of fresh or cooked vegetables or 1 cup of leafy greens.)
Best choices
Fresh or frozen vegetables, fresh vegetable juice
Acceptable choices
Canned vegetables, canned vegetable juice
Less preferable choices
Vegetables in fatty sauce; french fries and other deep-fried vegetables

FRUIT: 2 TO 4 SERVINGS PER DAY
(A serving is one average-size fruit, $^3/_4$ cup of juice, $^1/_2$ cup of canned or cut fruit, $^1/_4$ cup of dried fruit.)
Best choices
  Fresh or frozen fruit, fruit juice
Acceptable choices
  Canned or dried fruit
Less preferable choice
  Coconut

GRAINS: 6 TO 11 SERVINGS PER DAY
(A serving is $^1/_2$ cup of grain or cereal, 1 ounce of ready-to-eat cereal, or 1 slice of bread.)
Best choices
  Brown or wild rice; whole-grain and nonfat bread, crackers, bagels, muffins, pasta, cereals, pancakes, and waffles; air-popped popcorn (unbuttered); rice cakes
Acceptable choices
  White rice; whole-grain and low-fat bread, crackers, bagels, muffins, pasta, cereals, pancakes, and waffles; popcorn prepared in nontropical oils
Less preferable choices
  Fried rice; grains with fatty sauces; regular bread, crackers, bagels, muffins, pasta, cereals, pancakes, and waffles; buttered popcorn

---

Eight Great Healing Foods

While a balanced diet requires that you eat a variety of nutritious foods, some foods stand out as particularly valuable for the prevention and treatment of specific medical conditions. Here's a rundown of some of the best healing foods:

• **Apples:** They won't always keep the doctor away, but eating one a day should reduce your need to consult gastroenterologists, cardiologists, and oncologists. The pectin in apples helps prevent certain cancers (the pectin fiber binds with carcinogens in the colon and helps the body eliminate them), constipation (this soluble fiber acts as a laxative and stool softener), diabetes (pectin helps control blood sugar levels), diarrhea (the intestinal bacteria transform the pectin into a coating for the intestinal lining when irritated), and heart disease (pectin helps reduce blood cholesterol levels). All that and they're delicious, too.

- **Beans:** They help protect against heart disease (the soluble fiber helps eliminate cholesterol from the body), diabetes (the soluble fiber in beans helps control blood sugar), neural tube birth defects (due to high levels of folic acid), and osteoporosis (due to high levels of manganese).

- **Carrots:** Due to their high level of antioxidants, carrots—as well as broccoli and other vegetables—help to reduce the risk of many types of cancer, heart attack, stroke, and eyes disorders, among other medical problems.

- **Fish:** Among the most healthful fats are the omega-3 fatty acids found in a number of saltwater fish, including salmon, tuna, mackerel, sardines, anchovies, and herring. Omega-3 fatty acids help reduce the risk of heart disease by preventing the formation of artery-clogging plaque. They also lower rates of rheumatoid arthritis.

- **Garlic:** Allium compounds, found in garlic, increase the levels of certain enzymes that break down potential carcinogens. Allium compounds may also boost the activity of cancer-fighting immune cells. Studies indicate garlic helps prevent and treat stomach cancer, heart disease, high blood pressure, high blood cholesterol, and blood clotting.

- **Ginger:** Phytochemicals found in ginger help prevent cell damage that leads to cancer. Ginger lowers cholesterol levels and blood pressure and helps prevent blood clots that can lead to heart attacks and strokes.

- **Soy foods:** Soy foods—soybeans, tofu, miso, soy milk, soy protein, and textured vegetable protein (but not soy sauce)—have the same healing benefits as other beans. In addition, they contain chemicals—isoflavones and phytosterols—that help prevent cancer, especially breast, colon, and prostate cancer.

- **Tea:** The polyphenols in tea help prevent esophageal cancer; the caffeine and theophylline in tea helps to open bronchial passages during asthma attacks; the astringent tannins in tea help treat diarrhea; the manganese in tea helps preserve bone and prevent osteoporosis; and the fluoride in tea helps prevent tooth decay.

CHAPTER 8

৵

Shaping Your Body:
Tips for Successful Weight Control

Two out of three Americans are overweight, according to national surveys, and one out of three is obese (or more than 20 percent above their ideal weight). Over the years those extra pounds take a toll on overall health, contributing to heart disease, diabetes, high blood pressure, gallstones, and some types of cancer. In fact, experts believe obesity and weight problems contribute to more than 300,000 deaths a year. Fortunately, lowering your weight can lower your risk of developing these life-threatening conditions.

The Great Weight Debate

While all the experts agree that too much body fat is hazardous to your health, there is little consensus on how much fat is too much. Back in 1990 the federal government's suggested weight charts allowed for wide variations in weight. These charts also established a separate and more liberal set of standards for people over age 35, sending a clear message that putting on a little weight during middle age would not necessarily hurt you.

Not so, concluded the Nurses Health Study several years later. This fifteen-year study of 100,000 nurses found that the healthiest weights were 15 percent below the U.S. averages. In other words, it's not enough to not be fat; you need to be downright skinny to avoid a premature death.

Then, in late 1995, the federal government released a new set of guidelines that, as the table shows, falls between those extremes:

HEALTHY WEIGHT RANGES FOR MEN AND WOMEN
DIETARY GUIDELINES FOR AMERICANS, 1995

HEIGHT	WEIGHT IN POUNDS
(without shoes)	(without clothes)
4'10"	91–119
4'11"	94–124
5'0"	97–128
5'1"	101–132
5'2"	104–137
5'3"	107–141
5'4"	111–146
5'5"	114–150
5'6"	118–155
5'7"	121–160
5'8"	125–164

5'9"	**129–169**
5'10"	**132–174**
5'11"	**136–179**
6'0"	**140–184**
6'1"	**144–189**
6'2"	**148–195**
6'3"	**152–200**
6'4"	**156–205**
6'5"	**160–211**
6'6"	**164–216**

This table provides a good basic guide, as long as you keep in mind that the weights apply to all ages and offer a 30-to-40-pound range of acceptable, healthy weights for any given height. (Still, the upper end of the range on this table is about 10 to 15 pounds lighter than in the 1990 version.)

Another way to assess your weight is to calculate your *body mass index.* To determine your body mass index, multiply your weight (in pounds) by 705. Divide the result by your height (in inches). Now divide that result by your height again. Regardless of age, most healthy adults have a body mass index in the 20s. The risk of premature death rises as your body mass index rises above 25.

Whether you assess your weight using the height-weight tables or the body mass index, remember that the higher your weight or ratio climbs above the healthy range, the higher your risk of developing weight-related illnesses.

Location, Location, Location

Pounds alone don't tell the whole story. One critical issue is where those pounds are located. Fat around your middle—in the abdomen and chest—is much more hazardous than fat around your hips, thighs, and buttocks. (As a rule, it's also much easier to lose.) Abdominal fat enters the bloodstream more easily than fat from the lower body, raising cholesterol levels and increasing the risk of cardiovascular disease.

A quick look in the mirror can show you where you tend to pack on the pounds. Researchers have found that a waist measurement of more than 34 inches in women or 40 inches in men strongly correlates with other indications of obesity. If you want a more sophisticated assessment, you can calculate your waist-to-hip ratio. To do this, measure your waist (in inches) at its narrowest point; then measure your hips at their widest point. Divide the waist measurement by the hip measurement. Women should have a ratio of less than 0.8; men less than 1.0. A higher ratio indicates that you have too much abdominal fat and you should make an effort to lose weight, regardless of where your weight falls on the weight tables.

Get Moving

Of course, weight matters, but do not take for granted the importance of regular exercise. While researchers often focus on the link between overweight and longevity, recent research has demonstrated the critical role of exercise. Epidemiologist Steven Blair and his colleagues at the Cooper Institute for Aerobics Research in Dallas followed 25,000 men and found that among those who exercised regularly, the fat ones lived as long as the thin ones. And interestingly, the thin men who were out of shape were three times more likely to die than the overweight men who got regular exercise. In other words, exercise may be even more important than weight alone in determining who lives longest. Fat or thin, we all need to exercise regularly. (For more information on exercise, see Chapter 6.)

Exercise can also help you lose weight. Whatever type you choose, exercise increases your basal metabolic rate (the number of calories your body burns at rest), allowing your body to burn more calories even when you're sitting still. Studies have found that all it takes is 30 minutes of steady exercise to boost the metabolic rate for at least 12 hours. In addition, the muscle mass you build through exercise further revs your metabolic engine, since muscle burns more calories than fat, even when at rest. (A pound of muscle burns about 45 calories a day, compared to a pound of fat, which burns fewer than 2 calories a day.) While low-calorie diets can lower your metabolism, exercise can stoke your metabolism, making it easier to lose weight.

Exercise also helps you keep the weight off after you lose it. Research comparing people who lost weight through diet and those who lost through exercise found that the exercisers found it easier to keep the pounds from coming back. One study found that among people who kept weight off for at least two years, 90 percent exercised regularly (at least 30 minutes three times a week), and of those who regained the weight, only 35 percent were regular exercisers.

An Eating Strategy

If you need to lose weight, remember that weight loss should be slow and steady. If you try to drop more than a pound or two a week (either through diet or exercise), your body will switch into its fat-preservation mode and fight to keep you as plump as possible. Mother Nature designed us that way: Whenever the human body loses too much weight too fast, hormones cause the metabolism to slow down and hunger pangs to kick in to prevent us from wasting away.

Alas, there are no magic formulas or weight-loss secrets that will make the task of losing weight quick and painless. The truth (as you already know) is that to lose weight—and keep it off—you must change the harmful habits that made you fat in the first place. You must commit yourself to eating a well-balanced diet and getting regular exercise. That doesn't mean that you must swear off all of your favorite foods and become a martyr to the cause. In fact, drastic measures almost always fail. Instead, keep these tips in mind:

- Calories do count. While counting every calorie is unnecessary (and can make you nuts), you do need to monitor your calories rather than focus exclusively on fat intake. To figure out how many calories you can eat per day and lose about 1 pound a week, multiply your current weight by 10, then add 100 calories. For example, if you weigh 160 pounds, you can average about 1,700 calories each day and still lose 1 pound a week. Remember that cutting calories too much can undermine your diet by slowing your metabolism and making matters even worse.
- Fats count, too. If you want to lose weight, you need to watch your fat intake. (You should limit your fat intake to no more than 30 percent of calories from fat for your overall health, even if weight loss isn't your primary consideration.) Fat is calorically dense; you can eat larger quantities of food without increasing your calorie intake by eating low-fat foods. Feel free to choose low-fat or nonfat versions of foods, but keep an eye on your calorie intake when munching.
- Say yes to fiber. A high-fiber diet keeps the digestive system moving; it helps prevent certain types of cancer; and it fills you up, so you'll be less tempted to snack on less healthy fare.
- Add flavor to your life. Not with fat but with herbs, spices, and other seasonings. If low-fat foods taste bland and uninspired, punch them up with a trip to the spice rack.

- Don't forget the most important meal of the day. They're all important, but breakfast can be especially helpful in switching your body from the sleep mode into the high-energy mode. If you skip breakfast, you'll drag through the morning (metabolically as well as in mood), and you'll also be more likely to overeat later in the day.
- Don't skip meals. Breakfast isn't the only meal you should never skip. Skipping lunch or dinner can also cause your metabolic rate to drop. You will gain more weight if you eat a single 2,100-calorie meal each day than if you eat three 700-calorie meals. By spreading your calories throughout the day, you can actually eat up to 20 percent more calories without gaining weight.
- Don't get discouraged by the numbers. Some studies show that as many as 90 percent of people who diet and lose weight regain the weight—and often more— within five years. Before you lose heart, consider that these discouraging figures typically do not count people who lose weight on their own; instead, it measures those who turn to research programs and weight-loss clinics after repeated problems with losing. Successful weight loss requires more than meeting a certain goal weight; it requires establishing new diet and exercise habits. Without a permanent change in lifestyle, the chances are good you won't experience permanent weight loss.
- We all have our ups and downs . . . but try to keep yours to a minimum. Your body doesn't like to experience large fluctuations in weight, so it will strive to return your weight to its perceived "normal" point. After you lose weight, your body produces enzymes that encourage the regain of fat, and the fat is regained more readily with each major shift in weight. Some researchers suspect that this new fat tends to accumulate around the middle, the pattern associated with the highest risk of weight-related health problems.
- Lose weight naturally. A number of natural tech-

niques and products can be used to rev your metabolism and diminish your appetite, helping you to shed unwanted pounds. For specific information on natural medicine for weight loss, see "Obesity" (page 352).

CHAPTER 9

☙

Relaxing Your Body:
The Mind-Body Connection

Back in 1974 psychologist Robert Ader, M.D., Ph.D., set out to perform what at first seemed like a simple experiment: He wanted to teach rats to avoid drinking sugar water. Each time the rats drank a saccharin-flavored water in their cages, Ader gave them a dose of a drug that made them feel nauseated.

Then came the unexpected. When they were subsequently given sweetened water, many of the rats became sick and died—even when they did not receive the drug to induce nausea. Ader further investigated the drug he was using in his experiment and discovered that it suppressed the immune system, in addition to causing nausea. Ultimately he concluded that the rats had learned to voluntarily suppress their immune systems in response to the sugar water because they had established a mental link between sweet water and immune suppression. This landmark study was the first to demonstrate the powerful link between the mind and body.

The Role of Stress

Since the mid-1970s a number of studies have provided additional evidence for the link between the brain and the immune system. Scientists now better understand the hormonal and neurological relationships between the mind and the body, particularly the critical relationship between stress and immune function.

When faced with stress, the body kicks in to the so-called "fight or flight response," which involves a number of biochemical changes that happen in preparation for dealing with danger. In evolutionary terms this high-intensity state made sense when quick bursts of energy were required to fight off predators or flee a dangerous situation. Of course, in our own daily lives we face fewer of these life-or-death threats, but the modern world remains full of stressors— financial worries, health concerns, deadline pressures, relationship problems. When confronted with these contemporary stressors, our bodies respond in much the same way as our prehistoric ancestors once did.

In the body any stressor—either real or imagined—triggers an alarm in the hypothalamus in the midbrain. The hypothalamus then shifts into overdrive, warning the body that it must prepare for an emergency. As a result, your heart races, your breathing speeds up, your muscles tense, your metabolism kicks in to high gear, and your blood pressure soars. Your blood concentrates in your muscles, leaving your hands and feet cold and your muscles ready for action. Your senses become more acute: Your hearing becomes sharper, and your pupils dilate. You're ready to fight or flee.

As part of the intricate system of stress response, your body also releases adrenaline, epinephrine, cortisol, and other chemicals that inhibit the immune system and interfere with digestion, reproduction, growth, and tissue repair. While not harmful in short bursts, these stress responses can cause serious health problems if the stress continues for long periods of time. For example, someone working in a high-stress job or going through a difficult divorce might experience the physiological effects of stress for a prolonged period. Over the long haul these stress responses can contribute to the development of disease. Chronic stress can elevate blood pressure, contributing to hypertension; it can cause muscle tension, resulting in headaches and digestive disorders; it can suppress the immune system, leaving an individual prone to colds, flus, and a range of serious diseases.

Fortunately, the stress response can be quickly reversed. Your body begins to relax as soon as your brain receives the signal that the danger has passed and it's safe to calm down. About three minutes after the brain cancels the emergency signals to the central nervous system, the panic messages cease and relaxation begins. Your heart rate and breathing gradually slow down, and your other systems return to their normal levels.

Mind-Body Stress Relief Techniques

Just as your body can't tell the difference between the stress of a tiger attack and the stress of losing your job, your body can't tell whether the relaxation response was triggered by a change in circumstances or a change in your attitude. This can work to your advantage because you can learn to promote relaxation and reverse the stress response by using various mind-body techniques. Studies have shown that well-trained individuals have the ability to use mind-body techniques to voluntarily lower their blood pressure and heart rate, alter their brain-wave activity, reduce blood sugar levels, and ease muscle tension. With practice, you too can put mind over illness and use the following techniques to help improve your health.

Biofeedback

Biofeedback involves training yourself to use your mind to voluntarily control your body's internal systems. The technique has been successfully used to treat shortness of breath due to congestive heart failure, to assist in stroke rehabilitation, to help diabetics lower their blood-glucose levels, to lower blood pressure, and to relieve incontinence, among other applications.

Almost anyone can learn biofeedback, but it takes practice. It's easy to get stressed out but much more difficult to learn to relax and to control the precise effect of the mind on the body. To learn the skill, you must be able to measure your physical state. You attach electrodes to various parts of your body to measure your heart rate, breathing, perspiration, pulse, blood pressure, temperature, muscle tension, and brain-wave patterns. A small machine on the other end of the wires displays the data, usually in the form of pictures, graphic lines, or audible beeps. Using this information, you can literally watch yourself relax or grow more tense.

You can actually learn to control your body's internal processes by carefully studying the measurable changes in your body as you relax and change your thought patterns. Once you learn to adjust your physical state to promote relaxation, you can do it without all the equipment.

If you'd like to try biofeedback, ask your physician for a referral to an outpatient clinic, or look for a biofeedback center listed in the phone book. Before making an appointment, ask about fees and find out whether the training will be covered by your health insurance plan. For a referral you can also contact:

**Association for Applied Psychophysiology and
Biofeedback**
10200 W. 44th Avenue, Suite 304
Wheat Ridge, CO 80033
(303) 422-8436

Biofeedback Certification Institute of America
10200 W. 44th Avenue, Suite 304
Wheat Ridge, CO 80033
(303) 420-2902

Breathing

Deep breathing helps to relax the body and quiet the mind. Unfortunately, when they are stressed, most people don't breathe right: Instead of inhaling deeply and drawing in plenty of oxygen, they take shallow, rapid, weak breaths, filling only the top part of the lungs. This so-called "chest breathing," or thoracic breathing, fails to adequately oxygenate the blood, making it more difficult to manage stress, resulting in anxiety, panic attacks, depression, headaches, fatigue, and muscle tension, among other problems.

The preferred way of breathing is abdominal breathing, or diaphragmatic breathing. This type of breathing draws air deeply into the lungs, allowing the chest to fill with air and the belly to rise and fall. Newborn babies and sleeping adults practice abdominal breathing, though most adults lapse into chest breathing during their waking hours.

To relieve stress, become aware of your breathing and inhale more fully; you will immediately be able to feel the muscle tension and stress melt away in response to the improved oxygenation in your tissues. Concentrated deep breathing can help calm you and relieve stress at any time and in any situation. Of course, don't overdo it or you will hyperventilate. If you experience shortness of breath, heart palpitations, or a feeling that you can't get enough air when practicing deep breathing, stop immediately and return to your usual breathing pattern.

Controlling Your Emotions

When diagnosed with medical problems associated with aging, many people feel depressed, stressed, and angry—emotions that can make matters worse by further compromising the immune system. These feelings are to be expected, though you should try to take steps to work through them so that they do not further undermine your health.

Openly discussing the emotional side of illness can help many people resolve their negative feelings. Some people have success talking things over with a friend or loved one, while others need the assistance of a professional counselor or a support group for people who share a similar medical problem. For information on counselors or support groups, check the Yellow Pages or the social service department of your local hospital.

Massage

Massage is a hands-on way of reducing stress. The technique—which involves manipulation of the muscles, soft tissues, and ligaments of the body—stimulates blood circulation, slows the heart rate, and lowers blood pressure. It also stimulates the production of disease-fighting antibodies. Studies have found that massage reduces anxiety and stress-related hormones better than other muscle-relaxation techniques. And instead of making you feel drowsy, it can actually increase your alertness.

You can learn massage techniques yourself, either by checking out a book from a local library or by taking a class. You might also consider consulting a massage therapist, who should know a variety of techniques. Most states require licensing of massage therapists; if your state doesn't, look for a therapist with certification from a professional organization. For information on state licensing requirements and a list of certified massage therapists in your area, call the National Certification Board for Therapeutic Massage and Bodywork at (800) 296-0664. You can also contact:

American Massage Therapy Association
820 Davis Street, Suite 100
Evanston, IL 60201
(708) 864-0123

American Oriental Bodywork Therapy Association
Glendale Executive Campus
1000 White Horse Road
Vorhees, NY 08043
(609) 782-1616

Meditation

Though it comes in many different forms or traditions, meditation basically involves focusing your complete attention on one thing at a time. If you haven't tried it, meditation can be harder than it sounds: The mind tends to wander, and it can be a real challenge to maintain concentration when faced with a barrage of distracting thoughts.

Meditation relieves stress because it is impossible to feel tense or angry when your mind is focused somewhere else. You can't experience negative thoughts—or the physiological responses to those thoughts—if your mind is tuned in to a neutral stimulus.

Studies back up the idea that meditation promotes relaxation. Research done back in 1968 at Harvard Medical School found that when people practiced Transcendental Meditation (a type of mantra meditation), they showed physiological signs of deep relaxation: Their heart rate and breathing slowed, their oxygen consumption dropped by 20 percent, their blood lactate levels dropped, their skin resistance to electrical current increased, and their brain-wave patterns showed greater alpha-wave activity.

To experience the relaxing benefits of meditation, find a quiet place where you are not apt to be interrupted. Sit in a firm chair with your back as straight as possible, or lie down flat on your back on the ground. Then try one of the three basic types of meditation:

- Mantra meditation involves repeating—either aloud or silently—a word (such as *peace* or *calm),* a syllable (such as *ommmm),* or a group of words (such as *I am safe* or *It's okay)* each time you breathe out.
- Gazing meditation involves focusing both your attention and your gaze on an object such as a candle

flame, a stone, or a flower. The object should be about one foot away from your face. Gaze at it rather than stare, keeping your eyes relaxed. Don't try to think about the object in words, just look at it without judgment.

- Breathing meditation involves focusing on the rise and fall of your breath. Draw a deep breath, focusing on the inhalation, the pause before you exhale, the exhalation, and the pause before you inhale. When you exhale, say to yourself "one." Each time you complete a breath and exhale, count again, one through four, then start over with one. The counting helps clear your mind of other thoughts.

No matter which type of meditation you choose, begin your session with a few minutes of deep breathing. When random thoughts enter your mind during your meditation time (as they almost certainly will), don't become anxious; just accept the thoughts and let them pass through your mind without notice or response. Start by meditating for 5 to 10 minutes once or twice a day, then work up to 15 to 20 minutes.

For more information on meditation, refer to books in the library, or contact:

Cambridge Insight Meditation Center
331 Broadway
Cambridge, MA 02139
(617) 491-5070

Foundation for Human Understanding
P.O. Box 1009
Grants Pass, OR 97526
(503) 597-4360

The Mind/Body Medical Institute
110 Francis Street, Suite 1A
Boston, MA 02215

The Stress Reduction Clinic
University of Massachusetts Medical Center
55 Lake Avenue North
Worcester, MA 01655
(508) 856-2656

The Zen Center
300 Page Street
San Francisco, CA 94102
(415) 863-3136

Progressive Relaxation

Progressive relaxation can produce a profound feeling of calm, as you systematically remove the stress from your body. Start by lying on your back on the floor, with your legs flat and your arms loose at your sides. Close your eyes and breathe deeply.

Once you are reasonably calm, begin to systematically tense and relax every muscle in your body. Start with your feet: Tense the muscles in your feet for 30 seconds or so, then relax them, allowing your feet to feel heavy and relaxed. Then move on to your calves, thighs, abdomen, buttocks, hands, forearms, upper arms, shoulders, and face. When you finish, your muscles should feel soothed and relaxed. Lie quietly, and enjoy the feeling of complete relaxation.

Visualization

To relieve stress, use your imagination. Visualization—also known as guided imagery—builds on the idea that you are what you think you are. If you think anxious thoughts, your muscles will grow tense; if you think sad thoughts, your brain biochemistry will change and you will become unhappy. And more important, if you think soothing positive thoughts, you will relax and develop a more positive outlook.

To experience the relaxation of visualization, sit down in a comfortable position or lie on the floor in a quiet, dimly lit room. Tense all of your muscles at once, and hold for 30 seconds. Relax every muscle, and allow all the tension to drain from your body. Continue to inhale and exhale slowly and fully.

Once your muscles have relaxed, you can begin the visualization or imagery. First, concentrate on your breathing, feeling the regular rhythm of each breath and clearing your mind of all thoughts. Then imagine that you are in a peaceful setting, such as lying in the warm sun on a sandy beach or strolling down a country road on a cool October afternoon. Get all of your senses involved in your image: Smell the ocean mist, hear the leaves crunch under your feet. The more specific your fantasy, the more real it will seem. And the more real it seems, the more you will relax. Enjoy this "escape" for about 20 minutes. When you return to your body and get on with the challenges of the day, you will probably feel much more relaxed and refreshed.

You can also use guided imagery to visualize changes in your physical state. For example, if you have asthma, you might imagine your lung passages opening up, or if you have arthritis, you might visualize your muscles relaxing and your joint smoothly gliding through a full range of motion. The technique has been shown to help in the treatment of chronic pain, allergies, high blood pressure, and stress-related health problems. Many of the health benefits are directly related to the link between visualization and relaxation.

Guided imagery has also been used in the treatment of cancer. (Patients visualize powerful immune system cells consuming and destroying cancer cells.) While no well-controlled study has been conducted to prove the direct impact of guided imagery on cancer, studies have shown that the technique helps to ease anxiety and pain and to increase a patient's tolerance of chemotherapy and radiation treatment.

For more information on visualization, contact:

The Mind-Body Medical Institute
New Deaconess Hospital
Harvard Medical School

Boston, MA 02215
(617) 632-9530

The Academy for Guided Imagery
P.O. Box 2070
Mill Valley, CA 94942
(800) 726-2070

Yoga

Yoga promotes relaxation while at the same time strengthening and stretching the muscles. This form of exercise combines deep breathing with systematically moving the body into a series of postures, or positions. It can be very gentle and noncompetitive, making it an ideal exercise for people who have grown out of shape over the years.

But yoga isn't easy. It requires significant endurance, strength, and flexibility. Since it works every muscle group, weaknesses can be identified easily, allowing you to target areas that may need special attention.

For background on yoga postures and practicing the technique, check out a book on yoga from your local library, or take a class at local Y or recreation facility. Look in the Yellow Pages under "Yoga"; tune in to PBS for a nationally syndicated show, or try a video. Or you could contact:

Integral Yoga Institute
227 West 13th Street
New York, NY 10011
(212) 929-0586

PART THREE

NATURAL REMEDIES A TO Z

Alzheimer's Disease and Dementia

One of the advantages of growing older is that we accumulate the wisdom and precious memories of a lifetime. Unfortunately, Alzheimer's disease and dementia can rob us of this precious knowledge, which is part of what makes us who we are. Some four million older Americans—including two out of three nursing-home patients—suffer from Alzheimer's disease and dementia.

With Alzheimer's disease, the body malfunctions and gradually destroys the nerve cells in several key areas of the brain. As the disease progresses, the nerve fibers around the hippocampus—the brain's memory center—become crossed and knotted; these *neurofibrillary tangles* make it impossible to store or retrieve information. In addition to this internal short circuit, the brain also experiences a drop in the concentration of neurotransmitting substances, which further breaks down the body's communications network.

Dementia (or *senile dementia*) refers to general mental deterioration, including memory loss, moodiness, irritability, personality changes, childish behavior, difficulty communicating, and inability to concentrate. Alzheimer's disease is a type of dementia.

Alzheimer's disease, dementia, or any other progressive loss of mental functioning shouldn't be considered a normal or inevitable part of the aging process. These conditions are signs that something has gone wrong. In a healthy person intellectual performance can remain relatively uncompromised well into the nineties, provided the mind remains stimulated through learning. Most older people do not lose a significant amount of their mental functioning, and if they do, it is usually the result of a physical problem, such as a stroke.

Unfortunately, when it comes to Alzheimer's disease and dementia, we do not fully understand the disease process or what triggers it, though there does appear to be a hereditary link. What we do know is that the brains of Alzheimer's patients tend to have high levels of aluminum, calcium, silicon, and sulfur.

Alzheimer's is difficult to diagnose, in part because the only truly definitive test is a post-mortem biopsy of the brain. In fact, the disease is misdiagnosed as much as half the time at the first evaluation. Most of the people who are misdiagnosed are later shown to be depressed, which is not surprising since depression and Alzheimer's share many of the same symptoms in the elderly.

Words of Wisdom

"Everybody gets Alzheimer's disease. If it occurs at a young age, they call it Alzheimer's; if it occurs when you're 105, they call it the senility of aging, but it's all the same disease—the brain rots away from free radical damage. That's why everybody should take vitamins; long before you see evidence of Alzheimer's you should start to take vitamins and antioxidants. Vitamins can help prevent Alzheimer's, but there's nothing you can do to bring back brain cells that are gone."

Elmer M. Cranton, M.D.
Yelm, Washington

Conventional Care

When Alzheimer's disease or dementia is suspected, a physician should perform a complete medical examination, including a detailed history, physical exam, electrocardiogram, electroencephalogram, computerized tomography (CAT) scan, psychological evaluation, and neurophysiological tests to document the type and degree of mental impairment.

All of this information is necessary since four out of five people over age 60 suffer from a vitamin or mineral deficiency, which can mimic the symptoms of Alzheimer's disease or dementia. In addition, the workup gives the doctor a chance to consider other causes of mental impairment, such as a drug interaction (one out of three older people use eight or more prescription drugs every day), brain tumor, thyroid disease, Lyme disease (which can cause Alzheimer's-like symptoms), or high blood pressure (which can cause minor strokes that destroy brain tissue and cause memory loss).

Once diagnosed, a physician may prescribe one of several drugs used to control the symptoms of the disease, but these drugs cannot halt the progress of the disease.

The Natural Approach

All of the natural remedies listed below can be used to supplement conventional medical treatment.

Herbal Medicine

Use one or more of the remedies listed below. For more information on herbal medicine, see Chapter 2. Commercial preparations are also available; follow package directions.

- Alfalfa *(Medicago sativa):* This herb helps to improve blood circulation in the brain, which helps to oxygenate the cells and promote better brain functioning. To prepare an infusion, use 1 to 2 teaspoons of dried leaves (not the sprouts) per cup of boiling water. Steep 10 to 15 minutes, strain, and drink up to three cups a day.
- Club moss *(Huperzia serrata):* Chinese healers have long prescribed tea brewed from oriental club moss to reverse memory loss in older people. Since then, researchers have isolated natural compounds in the moss that improve memory retrieval and retention. To prepare an infusion, use 1 cup of dried moss per cup of boiling water. Steep 10 to 15 minutes, strain, and drink one or two cups a day.
- Garlic *(Allium sativum):* Animal research has shown that garlic appears to slow down brain deterioration of laboratory rats with Alzheimer's disease. Use garlic liberally in cooking; eat up to 6 cloves of fresh garlic daily; or use odorless garlic capsules, following package directions.
- Ginkgo *(Ginkgo biloba):* This herb improves the blood supply to the brain. Ginkgo is not generally available as a bulk herb, but it is available in commercial preparations; follow package directions.

Diet and Nutrition Supplements

Use one or more of the remedies listed below. For information on good food sources of particular nutrients and nutrition supplements, see Chapter 3.

- Coenzyme Q-10: This antioxidant, also known as vitamin Q, is produced by the body, in addition to being found in seafood and synthetic nutrition supplements. Take between 30 and 50 milligrams a day, following package directions. If possible, take the supplements with 1 teaspoon of peanut butter or olive oil (or as an oil-based capsule) to promote absorption.

- L-Carnitine: This amino acid provides the heart and skeletal muscles with energy by carrying fatty acids to the cells. It appears to slow the progress of Alzheimer's disease as well. Red meat and dairy products are best sources of L-carnitine, but since these foods are also high in saturated fat, supplements may be preferable. Take up to 2 grams a day.

- Vitamin B12: A deficiency in vitamin B12 causes symptoms that can easily be mistaken for Alzheimer's disease or dementia; even a mild deficiency can cause neurological disorders and memory loss. A vitamin B12 deficiency can also be caused by pernicious anemia. Vitamin B12 is found in meat, fish, chicken, and dairy products. Take a multivitamin containing 10 micrograms of vitamin B12.

- Vitamin C: This vitamin is a powerful antioxidant, in addition to helping to reduce aluminum levels in the body. Take up to 3,000 milligrams a day, in divided doses.

- Vitamin E: Vitamin E helps transport oxygen to the cells in the brain. Taken early enough, it may help to prevent Alzheimer's disease and dementia—or at least slow their progress. Take 400 IU a day; if signs of Alzheimer's disease are already present, increase the dose to 800 IU a day.

- Zinc: Even if you consume enough dietary zinc, your body may not absorb enough to perform all its necessary functions. Zinc is also an antioxidant, which helps prevent free radical damage that may contribute to Alzheimer's disease. Take up to 50 milligrams a day.

Homeopathy

Use one homeopathic treatment at a time, based on your specific symptoms. For more information on homeopathy, see Chapter 4. For dosage information, see pages 55–57. Discontinue use if the symptoms disappear.

- Alumina *(Alumina)* 30c: Use when confusion gets suddenly worse. One dose every 12 hours, for up to two weeks.
- Lycopodium *(Lycopodium clavatum)* 30c: Use when Alzheimer's symptoms include fear of being alone, insecurity, and frequent use of the wrong words. One dose every 12 hours for up to two weeks.
- Phosphorus *(Phosphorus)* 30c: Use when Alzheimer's symptoms accompany arteriosclerosis. One dose every 12 hours, for up to two weeks.

An Ounce of Prevention

Scientists do not understand fully the causes of Alzheimer's disease and dementia, but many experts believe that aluminum in the body can contribute to the development of Alzheimer's disease. To minimize your exposure to aluminum, avoid certain products (such as douches, feminine hygiene products, deodorants, and anti-dandruff shampoos containing aluminum), medications (such as antacids, some buffered aspirins, and antidiarrheal medications), and foods with certain ingredients (such as baking powder, pickling salts, processed cheese, and self-rising flour). At one time people were cautioned to avoid aluminum cookware, but research has shown that aluminum from cookware does not affect overall health.

New research also shows that supplemental estrogen may help to prevent Alzheimer's disease. Preliminary research indicates that women who take estrogen for two to three years cut their risk for Alzheimer's by about 10 percent. For more information on the pros and cons of estrogen replacement therapy, see pages 347–349.

Warning Signs

In the initial stages of Alzheimer's disease, the symptoms usually include forgetfulness, short-term memory loss, disorientation, moodiness, difficulty with mathematical calculations, and difficulty finding the right words. While many people fear they may be developing Alzheimer's, the fact that they are worried is a sign that they are not.

Alzheimer's disease involves more than mild symptoms. Anyone can misplace their glasses; someone with Alzheimer's disease might forget that they wear glasses. Anyone can get lost when traveling in a new city; someone with Alzheimer's can get lost inside their own house.

Often the symptoms seem to be worse at night.

In later stages of Alzheimer's disease and dementia, urinary and fecal incontinence, irritability, childish behavior, and violent outbursts are not uncommon.

For More Information:

Alzheimer's Disease Society
2 West 45th Street, Room 1703
New York, NY 10036
(212) 719-4744

Association for Alzheimer's and Related Diseases
70 East Lake Street, Suite 600
Chicago, IL 60601-5997
(800) 572-6037
(800) 621-0379

Alzheimer's Disease and Related Disorders Association
919 North Michigan Avenue, Suite 1000
Chicago, IL 60611
(312) 335-8700
(800) 272-3900

The American Journal of Alzheimer's Care and Related Disorders
470 Boston Post Road
Weston, MA 02193
(617) 899-2702

Caring for a Loved One with Alzheimer's Disease

Taking care of someone with Alzheimer's disease or dementia is a tremendous burden. It can be emotionally difficult even in the best of circumstances, but all the more so because the parent-child relationship may be reversed as the adult child nurtures and cares for the needy parent.

People who take care of Alzheimer's patients should contact the Alzheimer's Disease Society to receive information on managing the long-term stress of caregiving, as well as for referrals to local caregivers' groups. Individual counseling may also prove useful, so that the caregiver can have an appropriate release for the feelings of frustration, resentment, guilt, and despair associated with the challenges of dealing with a person with Alzheimer's disease.

10 Tips to Boost Your Memory

Having a good memory is like having a well-organized desk—the information is there, and you know how to get your hands on it. While memory-boosting techniques don't help much once someone has developed Alzheimer's disease, you can enhance your memory and your retrieval system by following a few simple tricks:

1. Pay attention. It's impossible to remember something when we experience sensory overload. Focus your attention on one thing at a time so that your brain will know how to file it away.
2. Make a mental picture. If you want to remember a name, take a "snapshot" of the person in context, paying special attention to what they are wearing, how they speak, and any other details that seem important to you. Try to focus on something distinctive about the person.
3. Make up a rhyme. To remember someone's name, make up a jingle or

rhyme associated with their name, such as "Anna Banana in a yellow dress."

4. Write it down. If you want to remember something, take notes. The process of writing will help you recall the information—and you will have written notes to refer to if, despite your efforts, you forget.

5. Say it again, Sam. (Your name is Sam, isn't it?) If you want to remember someone's name, repeat it out loud at least three times during your conversation. "Nice to meet you, Sam." If you want to remember something you read, discuss it with someone else.

6. Review to remember. If you want to remember something, review it soon after you absorb it. It may also prove useful to review the names of possible guests at a party or social gathering beforehand, if you're concerned about forgetting their names.

7. Cross-reference your files. Expanding on the idea that memories are stored in files, you can enhance your retrieval system by consciously filing a memory in several places. For example, if you want to remember that John's new baby is named Ella, you might want to remember that John's other child is named Hannah; both names have two syllables; both children have blond hair; as a child, you knew kids named both Ella and Hannah. Now, when you need to recall the names of John's children, you have several paths of retrieval; for example: childhood friend/two-syllable/Ella; blond/Hannah/Ella.

8. Make it easy on yourself. It's not cheating to use lists, calendars, pocket computers, and other tools to help you remember things.

9. Form consistent habits. You won't need to remember where you put the car keys if you put them in the same place every time you come in the door. Likewise, it's easy to find the car in the parking lot if you always park in the same general area when you go to the mall.

10. Use gimmicks. Try mnemonics to remember a list of items. For example, HOMES can be used to recall the Great Lakes: Huron, Ontario, Michigan, Erie, and Superior.

Anemia

If you feel tired all the time and get winded faster than you used to, don't assume the years are catching up with you. The symptoms you attribute to getting older may actually be caused by anemia, a condition in which the blood is deficient in either red blood cells or the iron-containing hemoglobin portion of those cells.

In the body the red blood cells transport oxygen from the lungs to the tissues and exchange the oxygen for carbon dioxide. If your red blood cells aren't up to the job, your tissues aren't getting enough oxygen. Fatigue and weakness are inevitable when your muscles, brain, and heart are working under such less than optimal conditions. You may even appear pale and washed out because your skin lacks oxygen-rich red blood. Iron also supports the function of many enzymes involved in the production of energy.

The most common type of anemia is iron-deficiency anemia, which primarily affects women. Iron is essential for the formation of oxygen-carrying hemoglobin. Iron-deficiency anemia usually shows up when the diet does not contain enough iron-rich foods or when the body fails to absorb the iron properly. As we grow older, our bodies become less efficient at using iron. In addition, iron reserves in the body may be depleted by blood loss, due to injury or internal bleeding (such as an ulcer), as well as by menstruation and pregnancy.

Anemia can also be a symptom of other dietary shortcomings, such as folic acid and vitamin B12 deficiencies. To diagnose the particular type of anemia and the most appropriate course of treatment, consult a doctor who will obtain a complete blood profile. Consider using natural remedies to treat the problem once it has been professionally diagnosed.

Conventional Care

If anemia is suspected, your doctor will probably perform a blood test to assess the composition of your blood, as well as to look for a deficiency in vitamin B12, a vitamin necessary for the formation of hemoglobin in the blood. If necessary, your doctor will prescribe iron supplements, in addition to encouraging you to eat a diet rich in high-iron foods. (Note: If you take antacids or calcium or zinc supplements, these should be taken separately from the iron supplements, since they can interfere with iron absorption.)

The Natural Approach

All of the natural remedies listed below can be used to supplement conventional medical treatment.

Herbal Medicine

Use one or more of the remedies listed below. For information on herbal medicine, see Chapter 2. Commercial preparations are also available; follow package directions.

- Angelica *(A. atropurphurea):* This herb helps boost red blood cell levels. To prepare an infusion, use 1 teaspoon of powdered seeds or leaves per cup of boiling water. Steep for 10 to 20 minutes. Strain, and drink up to two cups a day.
- Stinging nettle *(Urtica dioica):* This herb is rich in iron and other vitamins and minerals. For an infusion, use 1 teaspoon of powdered herb per cup of boiling water. Steep for 10 to 20 minutes. Strain, and drink no more than one cup a day.

Diet and Nutrition Supplements

Use one or more of the remedies listed below. For information on nutrition supplements and good food sources of particular nutrients, see Chapter 3.

- Iron: Make sure your diet contains plenty of iron-rich foods, such as liver, egg yolks, meats, whole-grain products, nuts, and seafood. If your doctor recommends, take up to 18 milligrams of iron a day. To avoid constipation, a common consequence of increased iron intake, drink additional fluids and increase your intake of high-fiber foods. Dessicated liver tablets are a natural source of iron, and you can get these in your local health food store. Or choose organic iron (aspartate, citrate, or picolinate), which won't constipate you. (For information on constipation, see page 221.) *Warning:* Keep iron supplements—and all nutrition supplements—away from children. Ingestion of iron tablets is a common cause of poisoning in children.
- Vitamin B12: A deficiency of vitamin B12 can cause anemia because this vitamin is essential for the formation of hemoglobin. Take a multivitamin with 10 mi-

crograms of vitamin B12, or talk to your doctor about taking additional vitamin B12 supplements.

- Vitamin C: To help your body absorb the iron found in plant foods such as vegetables and grains, drink orange juice and eat vitamin C–rich foods with meals. Studies have shown that you can nearly double your absorption of iron from plant sources by consuming vitamin C with the iron. If you choose to take iron supplements, consider washing them down with orange juice or another citrus chaser.

Foods to Avoid

If you have anemia, you should avoid foods and beverages containing caffeine, because it interferes with the body's ability to absorb iron. For the same reason, pass on iced tea, which contains tannins that also get in the way of iron absorption, as well as foods high in oxalic acids, including almonds, asparagus, beans, beets, cashews, chocolate, kale, rhubarb, and sorrel.

Homeopathy

Use only one homeopathic treatment at a time, based on your specific symptoms. For information on homeopathy, see Chapter 4. For dosage information, see pages 56–57. Discontinue use if the symptoms disappear.

- China *(China officinalis)* 30c: Use for anemia due to blood loss. One dose every 12 hours, for up to two weeks.
- Ferrum *(Ferrum metallicum)* 30c: Use when the face is pale but flushes easily. One dose every 12 hours, for up to two weeks.
- Natrum mur. *(Natrum muriaticum)* 30c: Use when anemia is accompanied by constipation, headache, and dry mouth and lips. One dose every 12 hours, for up to two weeks.

An Ounce of Prevention

As stated earlier, to prevent most cases of anemia, you should eat a well-balanced diet, including iron-rich foods. You might also consider using cast-iron cookware when preparing acidic foods, such as spaghetti sauce, since trace amounts of iron will leach into the food, boosting your iron intake. If you develop anemia despite eating well, consult your doctor to make sure you're not suffering from a more serious illness.

Warning Signs

Anemia offers some obvious warning signs, including pallor, tiredness, breathlessness, chilliness, depression, and heart palpitations. It can make people more prone to infection (especially thrush, an oral infection characterized by white eruptions in the mouth) and can cause women to stop menstruating. When anemia is accompanied by a deficiency in vitamin B12 and folic acid, a person can appear delusional and disoriented.

Anemia is particularly dangerous in people who suffer from atherosclerosis (a buildup of fatty plaque in the arteries that restricts blood flow). This combination of illnesses can severely limit the delivery of oxygen to the heart, brain, legs, and other tissues, leading to severe shortness of breath, chest pain, leg pain, and even stroke.

For More Information:

American Society of Hematology
1200 19th Street, N.W., Suite 3000
Washington, DC 20036-2422
(202) 857-1118

Franconia Research Foundation
1902 Jefferson Street, #2
Eugene, OR 97405
(503) 687-4658

National Heart, Lung, and Blood Institute
Information Center
National Institutes of Health
(301) 251-1222

Angina

The pain starts with constriction in the center of the chest, then radiates to the throat, back, neck, jaw, and down the left arm. You break into a sweat, struggle for breath, and feel nauseated and dizzy. You may assume you're in the throes of The Big One—a full-blown, chest-crushing heart attack—but within ten minutes or so, it's over, and the pain gradually subsides. What you've experienced is not a heart attack but a full-blown attack of *angina pectoris*.

Some three million Americans suffer from angina, a painful episode that occurs when the heart muscle does not get enough oxygen. (This is known as *myocardial ischemia*.) Most angina attacks occur when the heart, damaged by high blood pressure and coronary artery disease, is stressed by physical exertion, emotional upset, excessive excitement, or even digestion of a heavy meal. Attacks can be brought on by walking outside on a cold day, jogging to catch a bus, or hearing particularly distressing news. Angina attacks often serve as painful reminders that the heart has been damaged, and a full-blown heart attack may follow unless steps are taken to mend your ailing heart.

Conventional Care

Anyone with angina should be under the treatment of a physician. Your doctor may recommend that you take a daily dose of baby aspirin to prevent blood clots. (Do not start an aspirin regimen without talking to your doctor; even over-the-counter baby aspirin can have side effects and can interact with other drugs.) Likewise, your doctor may suggest a regular exercise program to improve your cardiovascular health. But work with a doctor or physical therapist to design a program that won't overly stress your already strained heart muscle.

In addition, your doctor may prescribe nitroglycerin tablets (nitroglycerin immediately dilates the blood vessels), beta blockers, calcium-channel blockers, or other drugs used to control angina. In some circumstances heart bypass surgery may be recommended to improve the blood flow to the heart.

Words of Wisdom

"A lot of homeopaths take pleasure in knowing that nitroglycerine—the great remedy for the heart—was actually derived from a homeopathic remedy. The homeopathic version is Glonoine: The 'gl' is for glycerine, the 'o' is for oxygen, the 'n' is for nitrogen. Back in the days when mainstream physicians set out to discount homeopathy, they discovered nitroglycerine—then they kept it as their remedy of choice."

Helen Healy, N.D.
St. Paul, Minnesota

The Natural Approach

All of the natural remedies listed below can be used to supplement conventional medical treatment.

Herbal Medicine

For information on herbal medicine, see Chapter 2. Commercial preparations are also available; follow package directions.

- Hawthorn *(Crataegus oxyacantha):* This so-called "heart tonic" helps in the treatment of angina and congestive heart failure by dilating the coronary arteries and improving blood circulation in the heart. For an infusion, use 2 teaspoons of crushed leaves per cup of boiling water. Steep 20 to 30 minutes, strain, and drink up to two cups a day.

Diet and Nutrition Supplements

Use one or more of the remedies listed below. For information on good food sources of particular nutrients and nutrition supplements, see Chapter 3.

- Carnitine: This vitaminlike compound helps the heart use oxygen more efficiently. Carnitine assists in the transportation and breakdown of fatty acids in the cells. Take up to 2 grams a day.
- Coenzyme Q-10: In the heart, coenzyme Q-10 helps prevent the accumulation of fatty acids; it also plays a critical role in energy production in the cells. Take up to 50 milligrams a day.
- Magnesium: A deficiency in magnesium has been shown to cause spasms of the coronary arteries. In fact, people who suffer sudden, severe heart attacks often have low magnesium levels. Take up to 250 milligrams a day.

Foods to Avoid

If you have angina or heart disease, you should avoid caffeine because it raises blood pressure and stresses the circulatory system. Likewise, limit your dietary cholesterol by switching to a low-fat or vegetarian diet and by increasing your intake of fiber, especially soluble fiber. If you do eat meat, choose only lean cuts, and limit intake to 6 ounces daily.

Homeopathy

Use one homeopathic treatment at a time, based on your specific symptoms. For information on homeopathy, see Chapter 4. For dosage information, see pages 56–57. Discontinue use if the symptoms disappear.

- Cactus *(Cactus grandiflourus)* 6c: Use when the chest feels constricted; when the person has difficulty breathing and breaks out in a cold sweat. One dose every 2 minutes, for up to ten doses.
- Glonoinum *(Glonoinum)* 6c: Use when the heart feels as if it is fluttering or throbbing; heat may make the symptoms worse. One dose every 2 minutes, for up to ten doses.
- Latrodectus *(Latrodectus mactans)* 6c: Use when chest pain is accompanied by numbness in fingers and a weak but rapid pulse. One dose every 2 minutes, for up to ten doses.
- Lilium *(Lilium tigrinum)* 6c: Use when the chest feels compressed and the heart feels as if it will burst; there may also be pain in the right arm. One dose every 2 minutes, for up to ten doses.

An Ounce of Prevention

Since angina is caused by coronary artery disease, particularly atherosclerosis, the best way to avoid it is to keep the heart and circulatory system as healthy as possible. A healthy heart requires a healthy body. If necessary, lose weight (see Chapter 8). Also, exercise regularly and follow a well-balanced diet (see Chapters 6 and 7).

Think of the pain associated with angina as the result of an artery-clogged heart starving for oxygen. Since smoking increases levels of carbon monoxide in the blood, thereby limiting the flow of oxygen to the tissues, smoking or being around others who do is one of the worst things you can do to your heart.

Warning Signs

Angina is a symptom of serious heart disease, not a disease in its own right. If you experience chest pains associated with angina, make an appointment with a cardiologist for a complete physical. During the appointment ask for specific recommendations on how to manage your underlying heart problem. (For more information on heart disease, see page 283.)

For More Information:

National Heart, Lung, and Blood Institute
Information Center
National Institutes of Health
(301) 251-1222

Anxiety Attacks

Anxiety isn't all in your head: It is also in your body, often expressing itself as trembling, sweating, a pounding heart, shallow breathing, confusion, a dry mouth, and difficulty speaking. We all feel anxious now and then, but uncontrolled anxiety or panic attacks can be debilitating and terrifying experiences, lasting from a few minutes to several hours or days. In some cases the episodes become chronic and ongoing, interfering with a person's ability to live a happy and productive life. While anxiety attacks can strike at any age, people often experience a growing number of anxiety-producing stresses in midlife and beyond.

Along with the physical symptoms, a person experiencing an anxiety attack typically feels an overwhelming sense of terror or impending doom. Unlike fear in response to danger, anxiety is an expression of a generalized, undefined fear. The physical and emotional symptoms are so severe and terrifying that people who experience anxiety attacks often end up in the hospital emergency room, convinced they are having a heart attack.

While there is considerable debate about the causes of anxiety attacks, many experts suspect that a neurochemical imbalance can trigger both anxiety disorders and depression. (People who are prone to depression also tend to experience anxiety attacks.) While some medications and psychological treatments can be helpful in managing anxiety and anxiety attacks, natural remedies can be used to minimize them by minimizing overall stress.

Conventional Care

If you experience chronic or severe problems with anxiety, seek professional help. Counseling and psychotherapy, as well as prescription antidepressants and antianxiety drugs, may be able to provide relief.

Words of Wisdom

"If you feel anxious, acupressure can help calm you down, slow your heartbeat, and let you think more clearly. Just rub the appropriate points while you do slow, deep breathing. You'll feel better immediately. With acupressure, you have relief right at your fingertips."

Shiva L. Barton, N.D., L.A.
Beacon Progressive Medical Associates
Brookline, Massachusetts

The Natural Approach

All of the natural remedies listed below can be used to supplement conventional medical treatment.

Herbal Medicine

Use one or more of the remedies listed below. For information on herbal medicine, see Chapter 2. Commercial preparations are also available; follow package directions.

- Garlic *(Allium sativum):* In the body garlic encourages the release of serotonin, a brain chemical that helps to regulate moods. High serotonin levels act like a tranquilizer to calm the nerves and relieve depression. For an infusion, chop 6 cloves of garlic per cup of cool water and steep for 6 hours; drink one cup a day.
- Skullcap *(Scutellaria lateriflora):* This herb helps relax the central nervous system and ease stress. To help calm the nerves, use 1 to 2 teaspoons of dried herb per cup of boiling water; steep for 15 minutes, strain, and drink up to three cups a day.
- Wood betony *(Stachys officinalis):* This herb is reported to have a sedative effect on the nervous system. Use 1 teaspoon of dried herb per cup of boiling water, and steep for 10 minutes, then strain and drink.
- Valerian *(Valeriana officinalis):* This herb contains chemicals known as valepotriates that have sedative properties. To prepare an infusion, use 2 teaspoons of powdered herb per cup of water; steep for 10 minutes. Strain, and drink one cup before bed.

Diet and Nutrition Supplements

Use one or more of the remedies listed below. For information on nutrition supplements and good food sources of particular nutrients, see Chapter 3.

- Calcium and magnesium: Taken together, calcium and magnesium have been shown to calm the nerves and reduce anxiety. Take up to 1,500 milligrams of calcium and 750 milligrams of magnesium each day.
- Selenium: Studies have shown that selenium supplements can reduce anxiety, depression, and fatigue. Other studies have found that taking selenium with

vitamin E or other antioxidants can improve mood and increase blood flow to the brain. Take up to 50 micrograms of selenium a day.

Homeopathy

Use one homeopathic treatment at a time, based on your specific symptoms. For information on homeopathy, see Chapter 4. For dosage information, see pages 56–57. Discontinue use if the symptoms disappear.

- Arsenicum *(Arsenicum album)* 6c: Use when the anxiety is accompanied by a rapid pulse, feelings of insecurity, and restlessness. One dose every 2 hours, for up to ten doses.
- Calcarea *(Calcarea carbonica)* 6c: Use when the anxiety is accompanied by depression, fear of insanity, and apprehension about being made a fool. One dose every 2 hours, for up to ten doses.
- Ignatia *(Ignatia amara)* 6c: Use when the anxiety follows the loss of a loved one or the breakup of a love affair. One dose every 2 hours, for up to ten doses.
- Lycopodium *(Lycopodium clavatum)* 6c: Use when the anxiety is linked to lack of confidence or fear of performing in public. One dose every 2 hours, for up to ten doses.
- Phosphorus *(Phosphorus)* 6c: Use when anxiety is accompanied by nervousness and generalized fear. One dose every 2 hours, for up to ten doses.

Acupressure

Use one or more of the acupressure points listed below. For information on acupressure, see Chapter 5. For diagrams showing the specific pressure points, see pages 88–91.

- Bladder 10: One finger-width below the base of the skull, on the ropy muscles a half-inch out from the spine.

- Conception Vessel 6: Two to three finger-widths below the navel, in the middle of the abdomen.
- Conception Vessel 12: On the midline of the abdomen, halfway between the navel and the edge of the breastbone.
- Conception Vessel 17: In the middle of the chest, in line with the nipples.
- Heart 7: With your palms facing upward, on the little-finger side of the forearm, in the hollow at the crease of the wrist.
- Pericardium 6: In the middle of the inside of the forearm, between the tendons, three finger-widths up from the wrist case.

An Ounce of Prevention

You may not be able to eliminate all anxiety or anxiety attacks from your life, but you may be able to minimize their frequency and intensity by getting exercise, practicing relaxation techniques, and using biofeedback to control stress. Be sure to eat a well-balanced diet, and don't hesitate to seek professional psychological help if you need it.

Warning Signs

Anxiety attacks can strike without warning. One minute you feel fine, and the next you panic and feel certain you're having a heart attack. If you experience anxiety or an anxiety attack, after you recover from the initial shock, take steps to understand what has happened to you and to get the support you need to prevent or manage any problems that may surface in the future.

For More Information:

Anxiety Disorders Association of America
6000 Executive Boulevard, Suite 513
Rockville, MD 20852
(301) 231-9350

Council on Anxiety Disorders
P.O. Box 17011
Winston-Salem, NC 27116
(910) 722-7760

National Mental Health Association
1021 Prince Street
Alexandria, VA 22314
(703) 684-7722

Arthritis: Osteoarthritis

Over the years your body shows certain signs of wear and tear. Outwardly you may have sprouted a few gray hairs, and your face may be creased with a few wrinkles. And inwardly chances are good that your joints have started to act up—the most painful sign of osteoarthritis.

Unlike other types of arthritis, which can strike suddenly, osteoarthritis usually takes its toll gradually, with the symptoms becoming worse over a number of years. Osteoarthritis afflicts, to some degree, approximately 40 million Americans—one out of every seven people—including 80 to 90 percent of people over age 50 and almost everyone over age 60.

This degenerative joint disease involves the breakdown of cartilage and bone in the joints, especially the joints of the fingers, hips, knees, and spine. In most cases decades of use gradually damage the cartilage in the joints, causing it to harden and form bone spurs. This cartilage breakdown causes the pain, inflammation, deformity, and restriction in range of motion characteristic of osteoarthritis. Osteoarthritis can also be caused by an injury, a trauma, a physical abnormality in the joint, or a previous joint disease.

In many cases the problem affects the *synovial joint,* a gel-filled capsule consisting of connective tissue that attaches one bone to another in a way that allows movement. To create a smooth hinge between the bones, cartilage covers the ends of the bones, and a membrane inside the joint secretes a lubricating gel known as synovial fluid. An outer shell or joint capsule surrounds the various components of the joint and keeps them intact. This system works remarkably well. In a healthy joint the bones glide back and forth and allow movement without grinding or rubbing bone against bone.

In a person with arthritis, however, the joint has become damaged or diseased. There may not be enough synovial fluid in the joint, causing stiffness, or there may be too much, causing swelling around the joint. If the cartilage at the ends of the bones has worn or chipped away, bone may scrape against bone, causing additional pain.

Conventional Care

To control their symptoms, most people with osteoarthritis turn to aspirin and other nonsteroidal anti-inflammatory drugs (NSAIDs). These drugs are available in both prescription and nonprescription strengths and can be very effective in controlling inflammation and pain—at least until the negative side effects become unbearable.

Many of the drugs commonly used to treat arthritis can actually promote joint damage. These drugs mask the symptoms, which can make you feel better temporarily, but they do nothing to manage the underlying disease. NSAIDs can exacerbate joint deterioration by inhibiting the body's ability to repair cartilage in the joints. The higher the dose and the longer the drugs are used, the greater the risk of additional joint damage.

For aspirin to reduce the symptoms of arthritis, it must be taken in high doses—often 12 to 20 tablets a day, depending on a person's size and weight. It can be tricky to keep the level of aspirin high enough to be effective, yet low enough to avoid overdose. In most people aspirin overdose first shows up as tinnitus (ringing in the ears). Other side effects of both aspirin and other NSAIDs include ulcers, bleeding, fluid retention, and decreased kidney function. To prevent damaging side effects, people taking megadoses of aspirin should be monitored by a physician, who can test the aspirin (salicylate) levels in the blood using a simple blood test.

Nonaspirin NSAIDs share many of aspirin's negative side effects, but they offer one major advantage: They are more potent, so you need fewer tablets to reach a therapeutic level. For example, 100 milligrams of one NSAID may be the equivalent of 1,000 milligrams of aspirin. On the downside, other NSAIDs tend to be considerably more expensive than aspirin.

Words of Wisdom

"Arthritis: It's inevitable once you're over 50, but it's a rather indolent process. Prevention is the primary key to limiting the disease process. Good nutrition—vitamins A, C, E, and other antioxidants—that's important, but if you want to avoid osteoarthritis, don't jog. Doctors' offices are filled with former joggers. Exercise is important, but choose low-impact exercise."

John T. Taylor, D.O.
Amarillo, Texas

The Natural Approach

All of the natural remedies listed below can be used to supplement conventional medical treatment.

Herbal Medicine

Use one or more of the remedies listed below. For information on herbal medicine, see Chapter 2. Commercial preparations are also available; follow package directions.

- Alfalfa *(Medicago sativa):* Alfalfa is often used to alleviate the inflammation and pain associated with arthritis. For an infusion, add 1 to 2 teaspoons of dried herb to 1 cup of boiling water. Steep for 15 minutes, strain, and drink up to three cups a day.
- Angelica *(A. atropurphurea):* Angelica's anti-inflammatory effects have made it a favorite arthritis treatment in Asian cultures for centuries. For a decoction, use 1 teaspoon of powdered root per cup of water. Bring to a boil, simmer 2 minutes, then remove from heat and let stand for 15 minutes. Drink up to two cups a day.
- Black cohosh *(Cimicifuga racemosa):* For centuries the Algonquian Indians used decoctions of black cohosh to treat arthritis. For a decoction, simmer ½ teaspoon of powdered root or 1 teaspoon of cut and sifted root per cup of water for 30 minutes. Cool, strain, and drink 2 tablespoons every few hours, up to one cup a day.
- Boswellia *(Boswellia serrata):* The gum resin from this large branching tree from India is used in the treatment of arthritis because of its anti-inflammatory effects and because it improves the blood supply to the joints. This herb is generally available only as a prepared commercial product.
- Devil's claw *(Harpagophytum porcumbens):* Devil's claw has both anti-inflammatory and analgesic effects; it contains a chemical, harpagoside, that reduces joint inflammation. For an infusion, add 1 to 2 teaspoons of dried herb to 1 cup of boiling water. Steep for 15 minutes. Cool, and drink up to two cups a day.
- Fenugreek *(Trigonella foenum-graecum):* This herb helps fight inflammation, making it useful in the treatment of arthritis. It also reduces cholesterol levels.

For a decoction, simmer 2 teaspoons of crushed seeds per cup of water for 20 to 30 minutes; be sure to cover the pot. Cool, and drink up to three cups a day.

- Juniper *(Juniperus communis):* This herb reduces inflammation and is prescribed widely in Europe for the treatment of arthritis. It is also used in the treatment of premenstrual syndrome and high blood pressure. For a decoction, use 1 teaspoon of crushed berries per cup of water, and simmer for 20 to 30 minutes. Cool, and drink up to two cups a day.

- Meadowsweet *(Filipendula ulmaria):* Herbalists have long recommended meadowsweet to treat arthritis; the herb contains salicin, the powerful analgesic and anti-inflammatory agent found in aspirin. For an infusion, use 1 to 2 teaspoons of dried herb per cup of boiling water. Steep for 20 to 30 minutes, strain, and drink up to three cups a day.

- White willow *(Salix alba):* Aspirin was first developed from a chemical derived from the bark of the white willow. This herb helps relieve pain and reduce inflammation. For an infusion, soak 1 teaspoon of powdered bark per cup of cold water for 8 hours. Strain, and drink up to three cups a day. If you don't want to wait that long, prepare a decoction by adding 1 teaspoon of powdered bark to 1 cup of water and simmering for 30 to 60 minutes.

Diet and Nutrition Supplements

Use one or more of the remedies listed below. For information on nutrition supplements and good food sources of particular nutrients, see Chapter 3.

- Boron: Boron is necessary for the formation and maintenance of cartilage, but it is not included in many multiple-vitamin, multiple-mineral formulas because the federal government has not established an RDA for boron. If you have osteoarthritis and your daily vitamin routine does not include boron, consider taking a supplement that provides 6 to 9 milligrams a day of the mineral.

- Glucosamine and chondroitin sulfate: As people age, their bodies produce less glucosamine and chondroitin sulfate, substances found inside the joints that help in the formation of cartilage. Without enough glucosamine and chondroitin, cartilage loses water and becomes a less effective cushion. Taking glucosamine-chondroitin supplements helps reverse the effects of osteoarthritis. Glucosamine-chondroitin combination supplements are available at health food stores and from some physicians. The standard dose is 1,500 milligrams (divided into three doses a day), but follow the directions provided by your doctor or on the product label. Be sure to pick up a product containing glucosamine *sulfate* rather than glucosamine *hydrochloride,* since the research on effectiveness has been performed on the sulfate form.

- Vitamin A, copper, and zinc: To produce collagen and cartilage, the body needs an adequate supply of vitamin A, copper, and zinc. Take a multiple-vitamin, multiple-mineral supplement that includes the RDA for vitamin A, copper, and zinc. High doses should not be necessary.

- Vitamin B3 (niacin and niacinamide): Studies have shown that vitamin B3 can be helpful in treating osteoarthritis when taken at high doses. Niacinamide and niacin are both forms of vitamin B3, but niacinamide appears to be better tolerated by the body. Still, niacinamide can cause liver damage at therapeutic doses, so vitamin B3 treatment should be used only under a doctor's supervision. Your doctor will perform a blood test every few months to monitor your liver function to protect against overdose.

- Vitamins C and E: Both vitamins C and E are antioxidants, which help prevent damage to cartilage in the joints, among other health benefits. Vitamin C also assists in the manufacture of collagen, a protein in cartilage. Without enough vitamin C, the body stops producing collagen, and the joints become compromised. Take up to 3,000 milligrams a day of vitamin C, in divided doses. Studies have also shown that vitamin E helps protect against cartilage breakdown, especially when taken in combination with vitamin C. Take 400 to 800 IU a day.

Foods to Avoid

Eliminating vegetables from the nightshade family—tomatoes, potatoes, eggplants, peppers, and avoiding tobacco—can promote cartilage repair. Nightshade vegetables contain high levels of alkaloids, which may trigger problems in susceptible people. The theory is that alkaloids remove calcium from the bones and deposit it in the joints, causing calcification, inflammation, and pain. An estimated 70 percent of arthritis sufferers who avoid nightshade-family vegetables report some relief from joint pain.

Homeopathy

Use one homeopathic treatment at a time, based on your specific symptoms. For information on homeopathy, see Chapter 4. For dosage information, see pages 56–57. Discontinue use if the symptoms disappear.

- Arnica *(Arnica montana)* 30c: Use when joint pain is made worse by an injury, such as overuse. One dose four times a day, for up to four doses.
- Bryonia *(Bryonia alba or B. dioica)* 30c: Use for severe pain that feels worse with the slightest motion. The pain improves with cold and feels worse with heat treatment. One dose four times a day, for up to four doses.
- Calcarea phos. *(Calcarea phosphorica)* 6c: Use when affected joints feel numb and cold; symptoms become worse during weather changes. One dose four times a day, for up to two weeks.
- Ledum *(Ledum palustre)* 6c: Use when pain involves small joints, such as toes and fingers; the joints may

crack and the pain may be relieved by cold treatment. One dose four times a day, for up to two weeks.

- Rhus tox. *(Rhus toxicodendron)* 6c: Use if joint pain is worst first thing in the morning or after a period of rest, then gets better with continued motion. The pain is relieved by heat but made worse by damp, cold air. One dose four times a day, for up to two weeks.

Acupressure

Use one or more of the acupressure points listed below. For information on acupressure, see Chapter 5. For diagrams showing the specific pressure points, see pages 88–91.

- Bladder 10: One finger-width below the base of the skull on the ropy muscles, a half-inch outward from either side of the spine. Relieves neck and back pain.
- Gallbladder 20: Just below the base of the skull, in the hollow between the two large neck muscles, 2 to 3 inches apart, depending on the size of the head. Relieves arthritic pain throughout the body.
- Large Intestine 4: On the outside of the hand, in the webbing between the thumb and index fingers, at the highest spot of the muscle when the thumb and index fingers are brought close together. Reduces inflammation and eases arthritis pain throughout the body, especially in the hands, wrists, elbows, and shoulders.
- Pericardium 7: In the middle of the inside wrist crease. Relieves pain in the palms of the hands and the middle fingers.
- Stomach 36: Four finger-widths below the kneecap and one finger-width outside of the shinbone. Relieves arthritis pain throughout the body, especially in the knees.
- Triple Warmer 4: Follow the outside of the arm to the hollow in the center of the wrist case. Relieves wrist,

forearm, and elbow pain; reduces wrist inflammation and improves wrist flexibility.

An Ounce of Prevention

To spare your joints, lose your spare tire. The more surplus weight you carry around, the greater the likelihood that you will develop osteoarthritis. Think about it: If you injured your knee, would you want to lug around a 25-pound bag of sand all day? To your knees, there's no difference between 25 pounds of fat and 25 pounds of sand. Losing the extra weight will improve your overall health in addition to reducing the stress on your weight-bearing joints. And of course, remember to follow the diet and nutrition recommendations listed above and to exercise regularly. (See Chapter 6 for more information on exercise; weight-bearing exercises, such as weight lifting, simple calisthenics, and isometric exercises can help to keep the joints mobile and the bones strong. In severe cases, consult a physical therapist to help design an exercise plan to meet your individual needs.)

Warning Signs

The first sign of osteoarthritis is usually joint stiffness, especially in the mornings and after long periods of rest. Other early symptoms include joint tenderness and slight swelling (inflammation is not common with osteoarthritis), cracking and creaking joints, loss of range of motion, and pain when the joint is used.

For More Information:

The Arthritis Foundation
1314 Spring Street, N.W.
Atlanta, GA 30309

(404) 872-7100
(800) 283-7800

National Arthritis and Musculoskeletal and Skin Diseases Information Clearinghouse
9000 Rockville Pike
P.O. Box AMS
Bethesda, MD 20892-2903
(301) 495-4484

American College of Rheumatology
60 Executive Park South
Suite 150
Atlanta, GA 30329
(404) 633-3777

Arthritis: Rheumatoid Arthritis

If you have rheumatoid arthritis, your body has turned on itself. This disease occurs when the immune system turns against the body and attacks the joints and organs.

Rheumatoid arthritis affects the entire body, causing chronic inflammation of many joints, as well as the skin, muscles, blood vessels, and in rare cases, organs such as the heart and lungs. If improperly treated, rheumatoid arthritis can lead to joint deformity. The disease causes the synovial membrane in the joints to divide and expand, causing inflammation and a buildup of joint fluid. Increased blood flow to the joints can cause redness and warmth.

In addition to joint problems, rheumatoid arthritis can cause fever, fatigue, weight loss, anemia, and tingling hands and feet. If the organs become involved, complications can include an enlarged spleen, irregular heartbeat, or pleurisy, an inflammation of the membrane covering the lungs. Lumps (called rheumatoid nodules) can also appear in the joints, especially in the elbow joints.

In some cases a person has a single bout with the disease, which then disappears and never returns (monocyclic rheumatoid arthritis). Other times the patient cycles between period of pain and periods of normal function (polycyclic). But in most cases a diagnosis of rheumatoid arthritis means chronic pain—and pain management.

The diagnosis of rheumatoid arthritis can be confirmed in about 80 percent of cases by a blood test for antibodies linked to the disease. Another test, measuring the rate of sedimentation of elements in the blood, can indicate inflammation in the joints. X rays can also confirm damage to the cartilage and bone.

The cause of rheumatoid arthritis is not fully understood. Some cases appear to be caused by a hereditary factor, but others may follow a viral infection. This serious condition plagues about seven million Americans, about three-fourths of them women. The first signs of the disease usually show up between age 35 and 45.

Conventional Care

To manage rheumatoid arthritis, most doctors use one of three types of drugs—nonsteroidal anti-inflammatory drugs (NSAIDs), corticosteroids, or disease-modifying drugs.

- Aspirin and other NSAIDs can be very effective in controlling the inflammation and pain associated with rheumatoid arthritis, though not without significant side effects. The drugs ease the pain and inflammation by inhibiting the formation of an enzyme that helps the body produce prostaglandins (chemicals that trigger inflammation). By cutting back prostaglandin levels, NSAIDs can reduce the redness, warmth, pain, and swelling associated with joint inflammation. But the drugs can also exacerbate joint deterioration by inhibiting the body's ability to repair cartilage in the joints. Other side effects include tinnitus (ringing in the ears), ulcers, bleeding, fluid retention, and decreased kidney function.

- Corticosteroids block the production of substances that trigger allergic and inflammatory reactions; this reduces swelling but leaves the patient more susceptible to infection and disease. Other negative side effects include increased appetite and weight gain, water and salt retention, high blood pressure, diabetes, thin skin, osteoporosis, cataracts, acne, muscle weakness, stomach ulcers, mental disorders, and adrenal suppression. Despite the side effects, some thirty corticosteroids are used, though on a short-term basis. They are primarily used when arthritis fails to respond to other medications.

- Disease-modifying drugs (also known as slow-acting or remittive drugs) interfere with the functions of white blood cells that cause joint damage. Others suppress the immune system by slowing cell division and making the entire immune system sluggish.

Words of Wisdom

"When it comes to rheumatoid arthritis, the treatment is very individualized. There are a lot of factors involved, but for most people there are natural things that can be done to minimize the pain. While it would be great if one treatment worked for everyone, it's really a matter of trial and error. Every person must experiment to find out what combination of treatments works best. Most people start out taking drugs, but they should not overlook the importance and effectiveness of natural treatments."

Susan Stuart, R.N.
Licensed Professional Counselor
Certified Health Education Specialist
Battle Creek, Michigan

The Natural Approach

Herbal Medicine
Same as for osteoarthritis (see pages 168–169).

Diet and Nutrition Supplements
Use one or more of the remedies listed below. For information on nutrition supplements and good food sources of particular nutrients, see Chapter 3.

- Fish oils: Omega-3 polyunsaturated fatty acids have been shown to relieve inflammation and the symptoms of rheumatoid arthritis. A Danish study of 51 people with rheumatoid arthritis experienced significant improvement in stiffness and pain after 12 weeks on a daily dose of 3.6 grams of omega-3 polyunsaturated fatty acids. (The amount used in the study is equal to about one 8-ounce serving of salmon, mackerel, or herring.) It can take three to four months for the benefits to show up from a diet that regularly contains fish. The most widely available fish oil is EPA (eicosapentaenoic acid), which is available in health food stores. Another type is DHA (docosahexaenoic acid); follow dosage instructions on the package.
- Selenium and vitamin E: Many people with rheumatoid arthritis have low levels of selenium, an important antioxidant that also helps slow the body's production of inflammatory agents called prostaglandins and leukotrienes. When selenium is taken with vitamin E, another antioxidant, studies have found that the supplements help ease the pain and inflammation associated with rheumatoid arthritis and may help stave off the disease in the first place. Most good multiple-vitamin, multiple-mineral supplements contain appropriate amounts of selenium (50 to 200 micrograms) and vitamin E (100 to 400 IU). Megadoses of these nutrients are not necessary.
- Vitamin C: The antioxidant vitamin C helps reduce inflammation associated with rheumatoid arthritis.

(For more information on vitamin C, see the section on osteoarthritis on page 170.)

- Zinc: People suffering from rheumatoid arthritis often have low blood levels of the antioxidant zinc. In addition to eating more zinc-rich foods, consider taking a supplement of up to 45 milligrams each day. Some vitamin-mineral supplements contain this level of zinc.

Fill Your Plate

The pigments that give fruits and flowers their color are known as flavonoids. In the body flavonoids have anti-inflammatory, anti-allergic, and antiviral properties, in addition to scavenging the body for harmful oxidants and free radicals. The flavonoids found in blueberries, cherries, grapes, and blackberries support the joint structures and collagen formation, so head for the fruit stand and start snacking.

It Could Be Something You Ate

Food allergies often trigger rheumatoid arthritis. Almost any foods can aggravate rheumatoid arthritis, but the most common are corn, wheat products, milk and dairy products, beef, pork, alcohol, nuts, and nightshade vegetables (see page 171). Food additives, dyes, and preservatives can also cause problems.

A reaction to a food can happen within minutes or several hours, and symptoms vary enormously. They can include diarrhea, vomiting, runny nose, rashes, hives, itching, and swelling in the lips, mouth, or throat. At the most extreme, food allergies can cause anaphylactic shock, in which the immune, respiratory, and circulatory systems react simultaneously, sometimes causing coma or death.

No single food allergen triggers arthritis pain in all people, so it's up to you to work through an elimination diet to identify an allergy, if you have one. It can be a long and tedious process to identify a food allergy. (The task is often made more difficult because many people are allergic to more than one food.) To do so, you should fast for two or three days (if your doctor approves), then introduce a new food every second day. If you notice an increase in joint pain or swelling within 2 to 48 hours, omit this food from your diet for a week, then try introducing it again. If your symptoms return, cut this food from your diet altogether. The process is time-consuming because it can take long periods to identify the offending foods. For additional information on elimination diets, contact a nutritionist. (See page 34 for tips on finding a qualified nutritionist.)

Homeopathy

Use one homeopathic treatment at a time, based on your specific symptoms. For information on homeopathy, see Chapter 4. For dosage information, see pages 56–57. Discontinue use if the symptoms disappear. In addition to the remedies listed below, see those included in the section on osteoarthritis, starting on page 171.

- Aconite. *(Aconitum napellus)* 30c: Use for severe pain and flare-ups in cold weather. One dose four times a day, for up to four doses.
- Pulsatilla *(Pulsatilla nigricans)* 6c: Use when joint pain seems to wander from joint to joint on a day-to-day basis. The pain is made worse by heat, and you feel weepy. One dose four times a day, for up to two weeks.
- Rhododendron *(Rhododendron chrysanthum)* 6c: Use when the pain is worse before a rain or storm. The pain often feels worse in hot weather. One dose every two hours, for up to two days.

Acupressure

See the listings under osteoarthritis on page 172.

An Ounce of Prevention

The cause of rheumatoid arthritis is not fully understood, so at this point there are no specific recommendations on how to avoid the disease.

Warning Signs

Rheumatoid arthritis usually first shows up as pain when moving a joint, especially early in the morning. It usually occurs first in the wrists and knuckles, or the knee and ball of the foot, though it can affect any joint in the body.

For More Information:

See the listings under osteoarthritis on page 173.

Bad Breath

Bad breath is easy to recognize—but its cause is sometimes harder to diagnose. One of the leading causes of bad breath *(halitosis)* is dehydration (the cause of most cases of "morning breath"). When we're awake, saliva works as a natural mouthwash, keeping the growth of bacteria in the mouth in check. But during sleep the flow of saliva slows considerably, and the pH of the mouth shifts from acidic to alkaline, allowing the bacteria to breed and let off that characteristic noxious sulfur odor. Other changes in the mouth's pH—due to fasting or eliminating carbohydrates from the diet to lose weight, for example—can lead to malodorous breath. Fortunately, the problem usually disappears following a thorough brushing, or after the saliva flow increases as the day wears on.

Periodontal disease causes many other cases of halitosis. The same bacteria responsible for gum disease let off sulfur compounds, giving your mouth a sour sulfur smell.

Treating the underlying disease will often eliminate the odor problem. Smoking, chewing tobacco, and drinking alcohol can also cause temporary bad breath.

Chronic bad breath, on the other hand, can be a sign of a more serious health problem, such as diabetes, kidney failure, cirrhosis of the liver, or certain cancers of the upper respiratory tract, which produce foul-smelling compounds. In rare cases foul-smelling breath can indicate a lung disorder, a gastrointestinal problem, or tuberculosis. Certain drugs, including some antihistamines, hormone therapies, lithium, and penicillin, may also contribute to bad breath.

Words of Wisdom

"Don't use commercial mouthwashes. They contain alcohol and artificial flavoring that can cause irritation, and they have no healing properties. Instead, use nonalcoholic mouthrinses found in health food stores. Look for products containing fennel, horsetail, white oak bark, or grapefruit seed extract. Remember, anything you put in your mouth is absorbed within 30 seconds, so put good things in there."

Dr. Harold Ravins, D.D.S.
Certified Dental Acupuncturist
Director, Center for Holistic Dentistry
Los Angeles, California

Conventional Care

Most episodes of bad breath can be effectively treated at home through improved brushing and the use of a mouthrinse to kill unwanted bacteria. Over-the-counter mints and sprays offer only temporary relief.

The Natural Approach

All of the natural remedies listed below can be used to supplement conventional medical care.

Herbal Medicine

Use one or more of the remedies listed below. For information on herbal medicine, see Chapter 2. Commercial preparations are also available; follow package directions.

- Chlorophyll: This herb freshens breath. Look for commercially prepared tablets at health food stores.
- Parsley *(Petroselinum crispum):* Due to its high chlorophyll levels, parsley eliminates bad breath. Either chew on a few stalks of the fresh herb, or take commercially prepared tablets.

Diet and Nutrition Supplements

For information on nutrition supplements and good food sources of particular nutrients, see Chapter 3.

- Buttermilk: Drink buttermilk and eat yogurt with active cultures to combat bad breath. These dairy products contain lactobacilli, which help fight off odor-causing bacteria.

Foods to Avoid

Some people who develop bad breath after eating garlic (as well as onion, broccoli, and other sulfuric foods) may have a deficiency in the enzymes required to digest sulfurous amino acids. To avoid producing the odor, avoid eating these foods.

Homeopathy

For information on homeopathy, see Chapter 4. For dosage information, see pages 56–57. Discontinue use if the symptoms disappear.

- Nux *(Strychnos nux vomica)* 30x: Use when bad breath is accompanied by a heavily coated tongue. One dose three times a day, for up to one week.

An Ounce of Prevention

Most cases of bad breath can be prevented by regular brushing of the teeth and tongue. Be sure to remove all traces of food that have been lodged between the teeth.

Warning Signs

While bad breath does not pose a health threat in itself, it can be a sign of periodontal disease or a digestive disorder. If you experience bad breath that does not respond to improved dental hygiene, consult your dentist or physician to rule out a more serious problem. (For more information on periodontal disease, see page 371.)

Cancer

Consider the odds: Every day our bodies produce more than 500 billion new cells. Every once in a while an error occurs, and our bodies form defective cells. This can be the beginning of cancer.

Cancer develops when oncogenes (the genes that control cell growth) are transformed by a carcinogen, or cancer-causing agent. In most cases the immune system identifies and destroys these aberrant cells before they multiply. But when the system breaks down, these fast-growing cancer cells reproduce, forming a tumor and invading healthy tissue. These tumors zap the body of nutrients and interfere with the tasks performed by the healthy tissue.

While cancer can develop at any age, it tends to affect older people more than younger ones because they have been exposed to more carcinogens over a longer period of time. In many cases it takes years or decades for cancer-causing agents to do damage; other cancers grow and spread rapidly. Some experts also speculate that older people may develop cancer more often because their immune systems become less proficient at detecting and destroying cancer cells.

While all cancers involve the uncontrolled growth of cells, the word *cancer* actually refers to more than a hundred different diseases. There are four main categories of cancer: *carcinomas* of the skin, mucous membranes, glands, and other organs; *leukemia* of the blood; *sarcomas* of the muscles, connective tissues, and bones; and *lymphomas* of the lymphatic system.

Not all tumors are cancerous: Benign (noncancerous) tumors do not spread and infiltrate the surrounding tissue; malignant (cancerous) tumors do spread or metastasize through the blood vessels and lymph system to other areas of the body, where new tumors grow. Areas of the body where malignant tumors most commonly develop are the bone marrow, breasts, colon, liver, lungs, lymphatic system, ovaries, pancreas, prostate gland, skin, stomach, and uterus.

Cancer is the second most common cause of death in the United States, after heart disease. Despite its prevalence, the exact cause of cancer remains a mystery, although some experts argue that environmental factors—such as exposure to tobacco smoke, radiation, asbestos fibers, and toxic wastes—cause about 80 percent of all cancers. In addition, some people may inherit a greater sensitivity to carcinogens and a greater propensity to develop cancer.

While many types of cancer can be treated—especially if detected at the earliest stages—the disease varies greatly in its aggressiveness. Natural remedies can help to bolster the body's defense mechanisms and restore its natural healing processes, but there are no "cures" that will work all the time. Consider the following natural healing techniques as supplements to your traditional course of treatment.

Conventional Care

Three main techniques are used to control the spread of cancer: radiation, chemotherapy, and surgical removal of the malignant tumor (and some of the tissue surrounding it). The overall success rate varies widely, depending on the type of cancer and the stage at which it is detected and treated.

Doctors differ in their approach to managing cancer, so be sure to consult at least two oncologists (medical doctors who specialize in cancer treatment) before beginning treatment. Some oncologists recommend very aggressive treatment, even when there is little hope of eliminating the cancer; others try to keep the patient comfortable and minimize the negative side effects of treatment when the disease is advanced and there is little reason to believe the treatment will be successful. This is a highly personal decision, and one that you should discuss openly with your family members and your doctors.

Words of Wisdom

"Cancer is not a disease, it is a symptom. The real problem is a weakened immune system. We all have cancer at the cellular level, but the immune system usually keeps it under control. To manage the cancer, you must strengthen and reeducate the immune system. Nothing is more brilliant or more dynamic than the immune system, nothing in the world—other than a miracle."

Bill Fry
Director, American Metabolic Institute
San Diego, California / La Mesa, Mexico

The Natural Approach

While natural treatments should not be used in place of traditional treatments, all of the natural remedies listed below can be used to supplement conventional medical treatments.

Herbal Medicine

Use one or more of the remedies listed below. For information on herbal medicine, see Chapter 2. Commercial preparations are also available; follow package directions.

- Alfalfa *(Medicago sativa):* Studies have shown that this herb can help neutralize some carcinogens. For an infusion, add 1 to 2 teaspoons of dried leaves to 1 cup of boiling water. Steep 10 to 20 minutes, strain, and drink up to three cups a day.
- Anise *(Pimpinella anisum):* This herb contains chemicals similar to the female hormone estrogen, which is sometimes used in the treatment of prostate cancer because it slows the growth of prostate tumors. For an infusion, crush 1 teaspoon of anise seeds in 1 cup of boiling water. Steep for 10 to 20 minutes, strain, and drink up to three cups a day.
- Apple *(Malus sylvestris):* The pectin found in apples binds with some carcinogens in the colon, trapping the dangerous chemicals and forcing their elimination from the body. In addition, the American Cancer Society recommends a high-fiber diet to prevent colon cancer. Eat an apple a day (including the skin, but skip the seeds, which contain cyanide).
- Black cohosh *(Cimicifuga racemosa):* This herb also contains chemicals that behave much like estrogen. (Due to its estrogenlike effects, it is used also in the treatment of menstrual and menopausal complaints.) For a decoction, boil 1/2 teaspoon of powdered root in 1 cup of water for 30 minutes. Cool, add lemon and

honey for flavor, and take 2 tablespoons every few hours, up to one cup a day.

- Dandelion *(Taraxacum officinale):* This herb contains a generous dose of the antioxidant vitamin A. A 1-cup serving of raw dandelion leaves contains 7,000 IU of vitamin A, more than one and a half times the RDA. Eat fresh leaves in a salad or as a vegetable.

- Garlic *(Allium sativum):* Studies have shown that garlic helps prevent stomach cancer. Use it liberally in cooking. To prepare an infusion, chop 6 cloves of garlic per cup of cool water and steep for 6 hours.

- Ginkgo *(Ginkgo biloba):* Ginkgo is rich in antioxidants that protect the body against free radicals, which damage healthy cells and can cause cancer. Ginkgo is not widely available as a bulk herb, but commercial preparations are available.

- Ginseng *(Panax quinquefolius):* Certain compounds in ginseng (saponins) have stopped the growth of some cancer cells in animal studies. The herb also stimulates the immune system. Ginseng must be mature and prepared properly for it to be useful; look for commercial herbs or preparations made from whole, unprocessed six-year-old roots. Follow package directions.

- Licorice *(Glycyrrhiza glabra):* Animal studies have shown that a component in licorice (glycyrrhetinic acid) can inhibit tumor growth. Licorice should not be used by people with high blood pressure; before using the herb, talk to your physician.

- Mistletoe *(Phoradendron serotinum):* For several decades, studies have shown that mistletoe inhibits the growth of tumor cells in laboratory tests. In Europe mistletoe-based chemotherapy agents are used in the treatment of lung and ovarian cancer. This herb should be used only under the supervision of a physician or qualified herbalist.

- Red clover *(Trifolium pratense):* For more than a hundred years, herbalists have used red clover to treat cancer. The herb contains several tumor-fighting compounds, as well as antioxidants. But it should not be used on estrogen-dependent cancers, such as breast cancer. For an infusion, use 1 to 3 teaspoons of dried flowertops per cup of boiling water. Steep 10 to 15 minutes, strain, and drink up to three cups a day.

- Saw palmetto *(Serenoa repens):* This herb is often used in the treatment of an enlarged prostate (benign prostate hypertrophy). By age 50, most men have a slightly enlarged prostate, which can cause either excessive urination or difficulty passing urine. Researchers believe the condition stems from excess buildup of the male hormone testosterone in the prostate, which is also linked to the development of prostate cancer. Saw palmetto reduces the impact of excess testosterone on the prostate, minimizing the risk of an enlarged prostate and prostate cancer. Saw palmetto is commercially available; follow package directions.

Diet and Nutrition Supplements

Note: To minimize the risk of developing cancer, the National Cancer Institute recommends that all Americans eat five to nine servings of fruits and vegetables daily, but only 9 percent of Americans heed this advice. According to experts at the NCI, as many as 50 percent of all cancers could be prevented by eating the right foods.

Use one or more of the remedies listed below. For more information on nutrition supplements and for good food sources of particular nutrients, see Chapter 3.

- Allium vegetables: Five hundred plants belong to the genus Allium, including garlic, onions, chives, and scallions. Use these vegetables liberally in your cooking. Garlic and onion are both rich in quercetin and selenium, two antioxidants that may play an important role in cancer prevention. Odorless garlic capsules are commercially available; follow package directions.
- Beta-carotene: This powerful antioxidant helps destroy cancer-causing free radicals in the body. Low blood levels of beta-carotene have been linked to an

increased risk of different types of cancer, especially breast, bladder, colon, and lung cancer. Eat a diet rich in high beta-carotene foods, and take a supplement of vitamin A of up to 10,000 IU daily. Foods high in beta-carotene include apricots, broccoli, cantaloupe, carrots, mangoes, peaches, pumpkin, spinach, and sweet potatoes.

- Calcium: Several studies have linked low intake of calcium with an increased risk of colon cancer. One study found that a daily intake of just 375 milligrams of calcium (approximately the amount in one 8-ounce glass of milk) was associated with a 50 percent reduction in the rate of colon cancer, while consuming 1,200 milligrams of calcium was linked to a 75 percent decrease in colon cancer. Researchers speculate that the calcium binds with fatty acids, preventing them from irritating the colon walls. A low intake of calcium may also increase the rate of excretion of vitamin D, which also appears to play a role in helping to prevent colon cancer. To enjoy these healthful benefits, drink two cups of nonfat milk or calcium-fortified orange juice, or eat two servings of low-fat yogurt daily. Take up to 1,500 milligrams a day.

- Coenzyme Q-10: Every cell in the body contains coenzyme Q-10, a protein that works with other enzymes to provide the cells with energy. Coenzyme Q-10 inhibits the formation of free radicals, unstable oxygen molecules that can cause cellular damage and cancer. It is commercially available in capsule form; follow package directions.

- Cruciferous vegetables: Epidemiological studies have shown that people who eat a diet high in cruciferous vegetables (such as broccoli, brussels sprouts, cabbage, cauliflower, and kale) have lower rates of cancer than people who don't. These vegetables contain indoles and sulforaphane, phytochemicals that help fight cancer. Eat at least two 1/2-cup servings of these vegetables every day.

- Ellagic Acid: Animal studies have shown that ellagic

acid, a polyphenolic compound found in fruit, counteracts carcirogens, preventing healthy cells from becoming cancerous. Eliagic acid is also an antioxidant, which blocks the negative effects of free radicals. Strawberries, grapes, and cherries are a good source of ellagic acid. Eat at least one 1/2-cup serving of these fruits every day.

- Fiber: Eat a high-fiber, low-fat diet to deter a number of different types of cancer, including breast and colon cancer. Studies have shown that women who eat wheat bran regularly have low blood estrogen levels; high blood estrogen levels have been linked to cancer. Eat 30 to 35 grams of fiber daily, an amount equal to at least five servings of fruits and vegetables daily combined with roughly six servings of whole grains.
- Flax: Studies have shown that people who consume diets rich in flax have lower levels of breast cancer. Flax contains an ingredient (lignans) that deactivates the estrogens that cause certain tumors to grow; these lignans bind to estrogen-receptor sites on cells in place of the more potent estrogens. Flaxseed oil is available in capsule and liquid form at natural food stores; follow package directions. Look for products with stabilized flax, since ordinary flax becomes rancid quickly.
- Folic acid: Studies have found that people who consume low levels of folic acid tend to have high rates of precancerous tumors of the colon and rectum. Take up to 400 micrograms of folic acid daily.
- Genistein: Genistein, an ingredient in soy and soy-based products, appears to prevent the growth of cancerous tumors by inhibiting the formation of the blood vessels that are necessary to nourish them. For example, studies show that the rate of prostate cancer is the same in Japanese and American men, but the cancers grow much more slowly in Japanese men, who eat a diet rich in genistein. Good sources of genistein include whole soybeans, tofu, soy flour, soy milk, and

rehydrated vegetable proteins (but not soy sauce). Eat one or two 3-ounce portions of soy foods per day.

- L-Arginine: This nonessential amino acid can stimulate the release of growth hormone produced by the pituitary gland in the brain. Animal studies have found that L-arginine helps inhibit the growth of tumors. Studies with human blood cells show that L-arginine increases the production of immune cells that interfere with tumor growth. Good food sources of L-arginine include brown rice, chocolate, popcorn, raisins, nuts, and sesame and sunflower seeds.

- Lutein: Lutein is found in fruits and vegetables in the carotenoid family; epidemiological studies have linked a high intake of fruits and vegetables rich in carotenoids with lower risk of cancer. Carotenoids give fruits and vegetables their orange, red, and yellow colors; they are also found in green leafy vegetables, although the color is masked by the green from the chlorophyll. Foods rich in lutein include broccoli, celery, collard greens, green beans, kale, peas, spinach, and turnip greens. Eat at least one serving of lutein-rich vegetables a day.

- Lycopene: Lycopene is a phytochemical found in fruits and vegetables in the carotenoid family. Lycopene gives fruits and vegetables their reddish color; it is found in red peppers, ruby red grapefruit, and tomatoes. Studies have shown a link between low blood levels of lycopene and increased risk of bladder and pancreatic cancer. Eat at least one lycopene-rich food daily. Commercial preparations are also available; follow package directions.

- Omega-3 fatty acids: In the 1970s scientists noticed that although Eskimos consumed large amounts of fat, they had an exceptionally low rate of heart disease and cancer. The fat in the Eskimo diet took the form of omega-3 fatty acids, which are found primarily in marine plant life phytoplanktons, which are eaten by fatty fish. A number of animal studies have found that omega-3 fatty acids delay the onset of tumors and decrease the growth rate, size, and number of tumors in animals in which cancer was induced. Good food sources include salmon, mackerel, albacore tuna, halibut, and sardines; eat two or three servings a week. While most researchers believe omega-3 fatty acids are most effective when consumed as foods, the fish oil is also available in capsule form. Take up to 1 gram of fish oil daily. Do not take omega-3 supplements if you are taking anticoagulants or taking aspirin daily, since excessive amounts of the acids can thin the blood.

- Quercetin: Quercetin is a bioflavonoid found in fruits and vegetables. Studies have shown that quercetin blocks cancer-cell development; epidemiological studies have also shown that people who eat a diet rich in onions tend to develop fewer gastrointestinal cancers. The best food sources of quercetin are broccoli, yellow and red onions, shallots, and zucchini. Eat at least one quercetin-rich food daily.
- Selenium: Broad-based epidemiological studies have shown that the mineral selenium may protect against certain cancers, particularly breast, colon, and lung cancer. Selenium inactivates peroxides in the cells, which can result in tissue damage. Dietary selenium is found in seafood, organ meats, and whole grains. Take up to 50 micrograms daily; most vitamin and mineral combination supplements do not contain selenium.
- Vitamin C: This powerful antioxidant has been shown to protect against breast cancer in postmenopausal women; studies have also shown that taking 3 grams of vitamin C a day reduces the number of rectal polyps, which have been associated with colon cancer. In addition, it appears to protect against stomach cancer by blocking the formation of nitrosamines, which are potential carcinogens. Take up to 3,000 milligrams of vitamin C a day, in divided doses.
- Vitamin E: A deficiency in vitamin E has been linked to breast cancer. It may also help to prevent stomach cancer and other cancers of the gastrointestinal tract

by inhibiting the conversion of nitrates in foods to nitrosamines, which are potential carcinogens. Take 400 to 800 IU a day. Do not take supplemental vitamin E if you are taking a blood thinner or have a bleeding problem.

Homeopathy

If you want to use homeopathy as a supplement to your regular medical care, contact a qualified homeopath. The following treatments can be helpful following breast surgery, if necessary. Use one homeopathic treatment at a time, based on your specific symptoms. For more information on homeopathy, see Chapter 4. For dosage information, see pages 56–57. Discontinue use if the symptoms disappear.

- Arnica *(Arnica montana)* 30c: Use immediately following breast cancer surgery. One dose every hour for the first 3 hours, then every 12 hours for the next three days.
- Staphisagria *(Delphinium staphisagria)* 6c: Use after breast cancer surgery if the healing is slow. One dose every 4 hours, for up to five days.

An Ounce of Prevention

While not all cancers can be avoided, taking steps to minimize your lifetime exposure to carcinogens can help lower your risk of developing some cancers. So steer clear of known carcinogens by living the clean life. Don't smoke; don't drink heavily; eat a low-fat, high-fiber diet; maintain your optimal weight; avoid unnecessary X rays; and check your home for radon gas.

To minimize your risk of developing skin cancer, limit your exposure to the sun. When you spend time outdoors—especially during the peak hours of 10 A.M. to 2 P.M.—wear a wide-brim hat, sunglasses, tightly woven clothing, and a broad-spectrum sunscreen with a Skin Protection Factor (SPF) of 15 or higher that blocks both UV-A and UV-B rays. Also wear SPF 15 lip balm; the lips don't contain melanin, and they are a common site for skin cancer. Avoid tanning salons; both UV-A and UV-B rays cause skin cancer, so don't fall for the hype that sunless tanning is safe.

Some doctors recommend taking one dose of baby aspirin every day to reduce the risk of developing digestive tract cancers (cancer of the esophagus, stomach, rectum, and colon). A recent study conducted by the American Cancer Society found that those who took aspirin were about 40 percent less likely to die from digestive tract cancers than those who did not take aspirin. However, do not start taking aspirin regularly without discussing the issue with your doctor. (Aspirin can also be used to help prevent heart disease; see page 287 for more information.)

And, of course, visit your doctor regularly for routine screening tests. (See Chapter 1 for recommendations on frequency of screening.)

Warning Signs

While many cancers grow silently in the body for months or years before making themselves known, there are some common symptoms of cancer to watch out for:

- a lump under the skin
- a persistent cough or chronic hoarseness
- coughing up bloody sputum
- difficulty swallowing
- chronic indigestion
- a thickening or lump in the breast (usually in the outer or upper part of the breast); there may be dimpling or creasing of the skin near the lump
- discharge from the nipple
- bleeding or discharge, bleeding between menstrual periods
- painful or heavy menstrual periods

obvious changes in bowel or bladder habits
blood in the stool or urine
a persistent low-grade fever
headaches accompanied by visual disturbances
fatigue
excessive bruising
repeated nosebleeds
loss of appetite and weight loss
change in size or shape of the testes
persistent abdominal pain
continuous unexplained pain in the back or pelvis
a sore or ulceration that does not heal
a change in a wart or mole; pay special attention to
  the ABCD rule:

- Asymmetry: Moles are symmetrical, cancers are not.
- Borders: Moles have smooth borders, cancers have irregular or poorly defined borders.
- Color: Variation in either shade or color from one area of the mole to another is a warning sign, as is the presence of red, white, or blue.
- Diameter: Moles larger than 6 millimeters (roughly the size of a pencil eraser) should be checked by a dermatologist.

For More Information:

American Cancer Society
1599 Clifton Road, N.E.
Atlanta, GA 30329
(404) 320-3333

American Institute for Cancer Research
1759 R Street, N.W.
Washington, DC 20009
(202) 328-7744

Cancer Information Service
NCI/NIH
Building 31
9000 Rockville Pike
Bethesda, MD 20892
(800) 4-CANCER

Make Today Count
P.O. Box 222
Osage Beach, MO 65065
(314) 346-6644

National Coalition for Cancer Survivorship
1010 Wayne Avenue, 5th Floor
Silver Spring, MD 20910
(301) 650-8868

Cancer Care
1180 Avenue of the Americas
New York, NY 10036
(212) 221-3300

People Against Cancer
604 East Street
P.O. Box 10
Otho, IA 50569-0010
(515) 972-4444

CANCER AND ALTERNATIVE MEDICINE

Atkins Center for Complementary Medicine
152 East 55th Street
New York, NY 10022
(212) 758-2110

Can Help
3111 Paradise Bay Road
Port Ludlow, WA 98365-9771
(206) 437-2291

Cancer Treatment Centers of America
Memorial Medical Center and Cancer Institute
8181 South Lewis Avenue
Tulsa, OK 74137
(800) FOR-HELP
(918) 496-5000

Committee for Freedom of Choice in Medicine
1180 Walnut Avenue
Chula Vista, CA 91911
(619) 429-8200

FACT—Foundation for Advancement in Cancer Therapy
P.O. Box 1242
Old Chelsea Station
New York, NY 10113
(212) 741-2790

Simonton Cancer Center
P.O. Box 890
Pacific Palisades, CA 90272
(213) 454-4434

Valley Cancer Institute
12099 West Washington Boulevard, Suite 304
Los Angeles, CA 90066
(800) 488-1370
(213) 398-0013

BREAST CANCER

Y-Me National Breast Cancer Organization
212 West Van Buren
Chicago, IL 60607
(800) 221-2141 Hotline M–F; 10 A.M. to 6 P.M. EST
(312) 986-8338

National Breast Cancer Coalition
P.O. Box 66373
Washington, DC 20035
(800) 935-0434
(202) 296-7477

American Society of Breast Disease
P.O. Box 140186
Dallas, TX 75214
(214) 368-6836

National Alliance of Breast Cancer Organizations
9 East 37th Street, 10th Floor
New York, NY 10016
(212) 719-0154

COLON AND RECTAL CANCER

American Board of Colon and Rectal Surgery
20600 Eureka Road, Suite 713
Taylor, MI 48180
(313) 282-9400

American Society of Colon and Rectal Surgeons
85 West Algonquin Road
Arlington Heights, IL 60005
(708) 290-9184

International Association of Colon Therapy
2204 Northwest Route 410, Suite 2
San Antonio, TX 78230
(210) 366-2888

United Ostomy Association
36 Executive Park, Suite 120
Irvine, CA 92714
(714) 660-8624

LARYNX CANCER

American Laryngological Association
Children's Hospital
300 Longwood Avenue
Fagan 9
Boston, MA 02115
(617) 355-6417

LUNG CANCER

Alliance for Lung Cancer Advocacy, Support and Education
1601 Lincoln Avenue
Vancouver, WA 98660
(800) 466-0701

American Lung Association
1740 Broadway
New York, NY 10019-4374
(212) 315-8700

National Heart, Lung and Blood Institute
Information Center
National Institutes of Health
(301) 251-1222

OVARIAN CANCER

Ovarian Cancer Prevention and Early Detection Foundation
P.O. Box 447
Paauilo, HI 96776-0447

PANCREATIC CANCER

American Pancreatic Association
Surgical Service, No. 112
VA Hospital
16111 Plummer Street
Sepulveda, CA 91343
(818) 895-9461

PROSTATE CANCER

American Prostate Society
1340-F Charwood Road
Hanover, MD 21076
(410) 859-3735

SKIN CANCER

Skin Cancer Foundation
245 Fifth Avenue, Suite 2402
New York, NY 10016
(212) 725-5176

Smoking: You're Never Too Old to Quit

One of the most common and most harmful environmental pollutants is cigarette smoke. This known carcinogen is directly responsible for most cases of lung cancer. Even secondhand smoke (or "passive smoking") has been shown to cause lung cancer and heart disease, as well as asthma and bronchitis in children.

In addition to causing cancer, cigarette smoke damages the lungs' ability to sweep out harmful bacteria, leaving smokers more susceptible to bronchitis and pneumonia. Smoking also causes chronic irritation that destroys the lung tissue, eventually leading to emphysema. Cigarette smoke also constricts the arteries, decreasing the blood supply to your legs, feet, hands, and skin (which can accelerate the formation of wrinkles).

The more cigarettes you have smoked in your lifetime, the more likely you are to develop these problems. But there is good news, even for smokers: When you stop smoking, your body begins to heal itself, regardless of your age. Within a couple of weeks your lungs begin to clean themselves. After quitting, every year that you do not smoke further diminishes your risk of developing health problems.

If you smoke, no matter what your age, stop. Of course, that's easier said than done. Smoking is one of the toughest addictions to shake, but about half of all Americans alive today who have smoked have managed to quit. Some people quit cold turkey, while others use the nicotine replacement patch. Whatever your approach, don't feel you have to go it alone. Support programs can make a crucial difference. The combination of lectures, behavior management techniques, and peer support is helpful. Low-cost or free programs are offered by many hospitals, as well as the American Lung Association and the American Cancer Society.

Cataracts

If you live long enough, the chances are good you will develop cataracts. This degenerative eye problem affects more than 90 percent of people over age 65. In fact, it is the leading cause of blindness in the United States, where at least two million people live with vision impairment due to cataracts and some 40,000 are blind due to the disease.

Cataracts occur when the crystalline lens of the eye grows cloudy or opaque. The lens, located behind the pupil and the iris, connects to the muscles surrounding the eye and flexes and bends as the eye focuses. As the eye ages, the lens gradually increases in size, weight, and density. Cataracts form when the eye loses the ability to maintain appropriate concentrations of sodium, potassium, and calcium within the lens, affecting vision. If your lens were a window, a cataract could seem like either a spot or a film of steam clouding the glass and obscuring your vision.

In most cases, the mineral imbalance in the lens stems

from damage caused by free radicals, due to exposure to ultraviolet light or low-level radiation from X rays. Cataracts can also be caused by disease, particularly diabetes, injury to the eye, a congenital defect, the use of certain steroids, or exposure to German measles during fetal development.

Cataracts don't always behave in a predictable manner. They can develop quickly or slowly; they can affect one eye or both; they can progress at different rates from one eye to the other. Cataracts aren't obvious in the early stages without the use of special instruments (the whitish film on the surface of the eye doesn't show up until the cataracts are quite severe), so regular eye exams are critical.

Conventional Care

When cataracts have become severe enough to impair vision significantly, surgery is the only way to restore sight. Fortunately, cataract surgery is relatively minor; it takes about a half hour and is performed under local anesthetic. Ophthalmologists perform about 1.5 million cataract operations a year in the United States.

There are several different types of cataract operation: *intracapsular extraction* (which involves removing the entire lens and much of the supporting capsule), *extracapsular extraction* (which involves removing the lens and a small part of the supporting capsule), and *phacoemulsification* (which involves shattering the cataract by blasting it with sound waves of special frequencies that do not damage other structures of the eye). Once the lens is removed, an artificial plastic lens is implanted to restore sight.

Words of Wisdom

"Prevention is key. Once a cataract has formed, it's very difficult to get rid of, even with natural medicines. I have seen some clearing with homeopathic treatments, but in most cases cataracts are extremely difficult to reverse.

Instead, I recommend that people prevent cataracts by consuming high amounts of antioxidants and by eating a wide variety of organically grown whole foods."

Thomas Kruzel, N.D.
Portland, Oregon

The Natural Approach

If you have already developed cataracts severe enough to impair your vision, don't expect natural remedies to reverse the situation. But you can go a long way toward preventing or halting the progress of the disease by following alternative treatments. All of the natural remedies listed below can be used to supplement conventional medical treatment.

Herbal Medicine

For more information on herbal medicine, see Chapter 2. Commercial preparations are also available; follow package directions.

- Bilberry *(Vaccinium myrtillus):* Bilberry contains bioflavonoids, which aid in the removal of chemicals from the retina of the eye. During World War II Royal Air Force pilots snacked on bilberry jam sandwiches before flying night missions to sharpen their night vision. Bilberry is available in capsule form from health food stores.

Diet and Nutrition Supplements

Use one or more of the remedies listed below. For information on nutrition supplements and good food sources of particular nutrients, see Chapter 3.

- Riboflavin (vitamin B2): Cataracts have been linked to a deficiency in riboflavin, a B vitamin that helps with metabolism. (About one out of three people over 65 are riboflavin deficient.) Take riboflavin supplements of up to 10 milligrams daily as part of a B-complex vitamin.

- Vitamin A and beta-carotene: Vitamin A and beta-carotene are vital for normal vision and can help prevent the formation of cataracts. Eat a diet rich in beta-carotene; a fourteen-year study of 50,000 women found that those who ate a diet rich in beta-carotene had a 40 percent lower risk of developing cataracts than those with a low beta-carotene intake. In addition, take a vitamin A supplement of up to 5,000 IU a day.

- Vitamin C: Studies show that vitamin C lowers intraocular pressure and helps halt the progression of cataracts. In addition, it protects the lens of the eye because it is a free radical scavenger. One study found that people who took between 300 and 600 milligrams of vitamin C had a 70 percent reduction in cataract risk. Protective effects appear with the intake of as little as 120 milligrams, the equivalent of 1 cup of orange juice or 1/2 cup of strawberries. If you choose, you can take up to 1,000 milligrams of vitamin C supplements a day, in divided doses.

- Vitamin E and selenium: These free radical destroyers work synergistically to protect the eyes. A selenium deficiency can promote the formation of cataracts; in fact, the selenium content in lenses with cataracts is only 15 percent of the level found in healthy eyes. Take 400 to 800 IU of vitamin E and 50 micrograms of selenium daily.

- Zinc: To retard the formation of cataracts and promote healing in the eye, take zinc supplements of up to 50 milligrams daily.

Homeopathy

Use one homeopathic treatment at a time, based on your specific symptoms. For information on homeopathy, see

Chapter 4. For dosage information, see pages 56–57. Discontinue use if the symptoms disappear.

- Calcarea *(Calcarea carbonica)* 6c: Use in the early stages of cataract formation. One dose three times a day, for up to seven days. If your condition improves, take one dose twice a day for two weeks more. If your condition does not improve, contact a homeopath.
- Silicea *(Silicea terra)* 6c: Use in later stages of the disease, when the cataracts interfere with sight. One dose three times a day, for up to seven days. If your condition improves, take one dose twice a day for two weeks more. If your condition does not improve, contact a homeopath.

Acupressure

Use one or more of the acupressure points listed below. For information on acupressure, see Chapter 5. For diagrams showing the specific pressure points, see pages 88–91.

- Gallbladder 1: In the slight depression level with the outside corner of the eye.
- Stomach 1: Directly below the pupil of the eye, in the center of the ridge of the bony socket below the eye.
- Stomach 8: At the corner of the forehead, one finger-width inside the hairline.
- Triple Warmer 23: In the slight depression at the outer edge of the eyebrow.

An Ounce of Prevention

To minimize your risk of developing cataracts, protect your eyes from ultraviolet light by avoiding direct sunlight and by wearing dark sunglasses and a wide-brim hat when outdoors. Since free radicals appear to be the leading cause of cataracts associated with aging, eating a diet rich in antioxidants can help protect the eyes.

Of course, regular eye exams are necessary to detect and treat cataracts in their early stages. Have your eyes tested by an ophthalmologist at least every five years. (An *ophthalmologist* is a medical doctor specializing in diseases and surgery of the eye; an *optometrist* assesses the need for glasses and writes prescriptions for glasses or contact lenses; an *optician* fills prescriptions for eyeglasses or contact lenses.) For a referral to an ophthalmologist in your area, check the Yellow Pages or call the American Academy of Ophthalmology.

Warning Signs

Cataracts tend to impair vision gradually, making it difficult to notice slight changes in vision. Regular eye exams are necessary to catch the disease in its early stages. Symptoms of more advanced cataracts include dull, fuzzy vision; glare in bright light (the cataract scatters the light before it reaches your retina); double vision; and changes in color vision (the cataract emphasizes yellows and reduces violets and blues). In addition, if you find yourself suddenly able to read without your regular reading glasses, get your eyes checked. This is a sign that your lenses are changing shape.

For More Information:

American Academy of Ophthalmology
655 Beach Street
San Francisco, CA 94109
(415) 561-8500

American Foundation for Vision Awareness
243 North Lindbergh Boulevard
St. Louis, MO 63141
(800) 927-2382

American Optometric Association
1505 Prince Street, Suite 300
Alexandria, VA 22314
(703) 739-9200

American Society of Cataract and Refractive Surgery
4000 Legato Road, No. 850
Fairfax, VA 22033
(703) 591-2220

National Eye Institute
Building 31, Room 6-A32
31 Center Drive
MSC-2510
Bethesda, MD 20892-2510
(301) 496-5248

To find out if your ophthalmologist is board certified, contact:

American Board of Ophthalmology
111 Presidential Boulevard, Suite 241
Bala Cynwyd, PA 19004
(610) 664-1175

Your Aging Eyes

If you're not wearing glasses to read this book, chances are good that sooner or later you will. As you get older—into your forties, fifties, and sixties—your vision will change, whether you've always had 20/20 vision or if you've worn corrective lenses all your life.

The official name for vision changes associated with aging is *presbyopia* (a term that actually means "old eye" in Greek). In youth the long muscle fibers in the eye contract or relax to alter the shape of the lens, allowing the eye to focus on objects near or far away. But as we age, extra fibers collect in the lens, gradually reducing its elasticity. This makes it more difficult—or impossible—for the eyes to change focus from near to far.

Fortunately, in most cases corrective prescription lenses can restore appropriate vision. Wearing glasses shouldn't be seen as a sign that your body is breaking down, but rather that it has been well used. Go ahead: Swallow your pride and get glasses. You will be able to see clearly once again—and you should be able to read the newspaper without holding it at arm's length.

Colds and Bronchitis

One advantage of growing older is that you're less likely to catch every cold that comes along. More than two hundred different viruses cause colds, and you must build immunity to them one by one. While drippy-nosed kids catch six to ten colds a year, most adults come down with only two to four a year. The older you get, the wiser your immune system gets about warding off the common cold.

A cold is a viral infection of the upper respiratory tract, which includes the nose, throat, sinuses, and bronchial tubes. When the virus invades, the nose and throat release chemicals to stimulate the immune system. As a result, the affected cells produce prostaglandins, which cause inflammation. In addition, the body temperature rises to boost the immune response, and the nasal passages produce more mucus to trap and wash away the virus.

When you have a cold, a battle is waged between the offensive virus and the defensive infection-fighting white blood cells. Surprisingly, it's not the virus itself but the body's defenses that make you feel lousy. In fact, the virus has been in your body for about twenty-four hours before you begin to feel you're coming down with a cold.

Bronchitis, an infection of the bronchial tubes in the upper part of the lungs, sometimes follows a cold. It can be the result of the virus, or a secondary bacterial infection. With bronchitis, you suffer from an intense version of the classic cold symptoms, plus muscle aches and fatigue. Since the bronchial tubes swell and fill with mucus, breathing also may be difficult.

Since viruses cause colds—and antibiotics don't work against viruses—when you come down with a cold, the best you can do is try to treat the symptoms. Colds are self-limiting: They last about a week, no matter what you do. All you can really do is treat your symptoms and wait patiently for the virus to be overpowered by the immune system.

The flu is the evil cousin of the common cold. Like a cold, influenza causes cough, fever, sore throat, and runny nose—but the symptoms tend to be much more severe. Add to the list of symptoms chills, exhaustion, red eyes, and muscle aches. To top it off, some people also experience nausea, vomiting, and diarrhea. While colds affect the upper respiratory system, flu also involves the bronchial tubes and lungs.

Unfortunately, there's nothing you can do but treat the symptoms and allow the virus to runs its course. Although antibiotics won't kill viruses, they may be needed if you develop pneumonia, strep throat, or some other secondary infection. Unless complications arise, you'll have to try to manage your symptoms one by one. Fortunately, there are a number of natural remedies that can help.

Conventional Care

The common cold can be treated without medical supervision, unless it develops into a secondary bacterial infection such as pneumonia (for more information, see page 377). As long as the symptoms are mild—albeit irritating—treat your cold at home. Get plenty of rest; drink plenty of fluids to prevent dehydration and to thin nasal mucus; and have some warm soup or hot tea to help relieve congestion and to soothe your sore throat. (Yes, chicken soup is more effective than water at clearing nasal mucus, according to a study conducted at Mt. Sinai Hospital in Miami Beach.)

In terms of medicating a cold, deal with each symptom separately. Avoid over-the-counter, multiaction cold treatments because they tend to overmedicate by giving you drugs to control symptoms you may not have. (Most cold symptoms occur serially, not simultaneously.) Instead, deal with the symptoms one by one.

Since influenza is caused by a virus, there's no way to "cure" it; you must endure the symptoms, while taking whatever steps you can to minimize them. Take acetaminophen or aspirin to lower the fever and ease the aches and pains. Use a humidifier to vaporize the air to make breathing easier at night. And drink plenty of fluids, including water, clear soups, gelatin, diluted fruit juice, and flat soda.

Words of Wisdom

"When you have a cold, the acupressure points on the neck tend to be key points. A cold is considered a 'wind' condition; you want to try to stop the wind from rushing into the body."

Lisa Wong, L.Ac.
Diplomate of the National Commission
for the Certification of Acupuncture
Agoura Hills, California

Natural Remedies

All of the natural remedies listed below can be used to supplement conventional medical treatment.

Herbal Medicine

Use one or more of the remedies listed below. For more information on herbal medicine, see Chapter 2. Commercial preparations are also available; follow package directions.

- Boneset *(Eupatorium perfoliatum):* This herb promotes sweating, which can help reduce fever; it is particularly effective for hot feverish colds and flu with muscle pain. For an infusion, use 1 to 2 teaspoons of dried leaves per cup of boiling water. Steep 10 to 15 minutes, strain, and drink up to three cups a day.
- Chamomile *(Matricaria chamomilla):* Tea made of chamomile will help you rest and relax. Use 1 teaspoon of dried herb per cup of boiling water. Steep for 10 minutes, strain, and drink up to three cups a day.
- Echinacea *(Echinacea angustifolia):* This herb boosts the immune system and helps fight viral infections. Take one dose of commercially prepared echinacea once a day, or as directed on the package label.
- Garlic *(Allium sativum):* This herb has antimicrobial and antifungal properties, in addition to helping to fight many different types of infection. Eat up to 6 cloves of fresh garlic a day, or use an odorless commercial preparation, following package directions.
- Licorice *(Glycyrrhiza glabra):* Tea made of licorice soothes a sore throat and helps relieve coughs. Use 1 teaspoon of dried herb per cup of boiling water. Steep for 10 minutes, strain, and drink up to three cups a day.

Diet and Nutrition Supplements

Use one or more of the remedies listed below. For information on nutrition supplements and good food sources of particular nutrients, see Chapter 3.

- Vitamin A: This vitamin boosts the immune system and helps fight infection. The vitamin A in a complete multivitamin supplement should provide an adequate dose.

- Vitamin C: This famous cold-fighting vitamin really can help reduce inflammation and boost the immune system. Take 1,500 to 3,000 milligrams of vitamin C once a day, in divided doses, beginning at the first hint of cold symptoms.
- Zinc: To boost the immune system and help fight off certain common cold viruses, suck on zinc lozenges throughout the day. Follow package directions for dosage information, or take up to 50 milligrams a day.

Homeopathy

Use one homeopathic treatment at a time, based on your specific symptoms. For information on homeopathy, see Chapter 4. For dosage information, see pages 56–57. Discontinue use if the symptoms disappear.

- Aconite. *(Aconitum napellus)* 30c: Use if sneezing, burning throat, and other cold symptoms develop suddenly, especially after exposure to cold. One dose every 2 hours, for up to four doses.
- Allium *(Allium cepa)* 12x or 6c: Use if a very runny nose and nasal inflammation accompany a cold. One dose three times daily, for three days.
- Arsenicum *(Arsenicum album)* 30x or 9c: Use if flu symptoms include weakness, restlessness, and chills. One dose four times a day, for up to three days.
- Eupatorium *(Eupatorium perfoliatum)* 12x or 6c: Use if flu symptoms include achiness and fatigue. One dose three to four times a day, for up to three days.
- Euphrasia *(Euphrasia officinalis)* 12x: Use if cold symptoms include irritated and burning eyes, especially at night. One dose three times daily, for three days.
- Ferrum phos. *(Ferrum phosphoricum)* 6c: Use when flu comes on slowly, accompanied by sore throat and mild fever. One dose every 2 hours, for up to four doses.

- Gelsemium *(Gelsemium sempervirens)* 30x or 9c: Use if fatigue and heavy eyes accompany other cold symptoms. One dose three times daily, for three days.
- Mercurius *(Mercurius solubilis hahnemanni)* 12x or 6c: Use if flu symptoms linger, accompanied by sore throat and tender swollen glands. One dose three times a day, for up to three days.
- Nux *(Strychnos nux vomica)* 6c: Use when flu symptoms include chills, runny nose, watery eyes, sneezing, headaches, and sore throat. One dose every 2 hours, for up to four doses.
- Pulsatilla *(Pulsatilla nigricans)* 6c: Use when nasal mucus is yellow and nose is blocked at night and runny during the day. One dose every 2 hours, for up to four doses.

Acupressure

Use one or more of the acupressure points listed below. For information on acupressure, see Chapter 5. For diagrams showing the specific pressure points, see pages 88–91.

- Bladder 2: In the indentations of the eye sockets, on either side of where the bridge of the nose meets the ridge of the eyebrows.
- Conception Vessel 22: Just above the breastbone, in the depression below the throat.
- Gallbladder 20: At the back of the head, in the depression between the bottom of the skull and the neck muscles.
- Governing Vessel 16: In the center of the back of the head, in the large hollow under the base of the skull.
- Large Intestine 4: At the highest spot of the muscle on the back of the hand that protrudes when the thumb and index finger are close together.
- Lung 5: On the inside of the elbow, in the hollow on the outer edge of the tendons, when the elbow is slightly bent.

- Stomach 3: At the bottom of the cheekbone, directly below the pupil.
- Triple Warmer 15: On the shoulders, midway between the base of the neck and the outside of the shoulders, a half-inch below the top of the shoulders.

An Ounce of Prevention

You can't avoid every cold, but regular hand washing can minimize your risk of coming down with every bug that's being passed around. Take steps to keep your hands away from your nose and eyes; a virus placed at the base of the nose can be inhaled up into the nose, where it can cause a cold. (Studies show most people touch their noses or eyes at least once every three hours.) If you can break the touching habit, you can dramatically cut the number of colds you get each year.

A cold is most infectious during the first three days after symptoms appear, so avoid people who are in the early stages of a cold. Keep in mind that cold viruses can live for several hours after being spread by a sneeze or cough. In addition, the stronger your immune system, the more likely you will be able to resist a cold, so eat a well-balanced diet and get plenty of rest and exercise.

To avoid the flu, consider getting a flu shot, especially if you are over age 65 or if you have chronic lung disease, heart disease, diabetes, metabolic disorders, anemia, or immune system illness. The vaccine helps fight the current influenza strain, though the shot itself can cause mild flu-like symptoms, including low-grade fever and minor aches.

Only about half the people who need flu shots actually get them. As a result, more than 20,000 Americans—mostly older people—die from influenza each year. Flu takes a greater toll on older people than the general population because they are more likely to develop complications, such as pneumonia and dehydration. However, flu shots are not for everyone. You should not get a flu shot if you are allergic to eggs, since the virus in the vaccine is grown in eggs, which can cause an allergic reaction in sensitive people. Talk to your doctor about other medications that can be used for short-term protection during flu outbreaks.

Warning Signs

Most colds start with a runny nose and a stuffy-head feeling. You're actually sick before you start to feel any symptoms, and there's almost nothing you can do but wait, once a cold virus has decided to take up residence in your nasal passages. If you experience sinus pain and congestion that doesn't clear up within ten days, call the doctor. The blocked nasal passages may have created a sinus infection, which should be treated with prescription antibiotics.

If you come down with the flu, the characteristic fever, headache, achiness, and fatigue will let you know it. If symptoms linger, if you develop difficulty breathing, or if a lingering cough follows the flu, contact your doctor, because a run-of-the-mill bout with the flu may evolve into a more serious illness, such as pneumonia.

Constipation

It could be caused by something you ate—or didn't eat. It could be a side effect of a new medication, or your body's rebellion to stress or travel. Whatever the cause, constipation can be difficult—and painful—to live with no matter what your age.

Constipation is not defined by frequency of bowel movements. In fact, when it comes to bowel movements, there is no single definition of normal. Some people have three bowel movements a day, others have three per week, but neither group is considered to have a problem as long as the stools are soft enough to pass without difficulty. In general, the body excretes waste in 18 to 24 hours (with a high-fiber diet) or 48 hours (with a low-fiber diet).

Constipation involves straining to pass dry, hard stools; it can also include gas pains and bloating. In severe cases, it can cause the digestive system to grind to a halt, resulting in an impacted bowel.

Constipation is common, especially among older people. As we grow older, the digestive system tends to become a bit sluggish. The problem can be made even worse by some prescription drugs (especially diuretics, antidepressants, antacids, painkillers, tranquilizers, iron supplements, muscle relaxants, anti-Parkinsonism drugs, and antihistamines).

Untreated, constipation can lead to hemorrhoids, headaches, varicose veins, indigestion, and possibly even bowel cancer. In addition, straining during bowel movements can create such pressure against the wall of the colon that the tissue becomes distended, forming pouches (known as diverticula) along the colon, which stretch and fill with stool. The pouches can be quite painful, causing abdominal cramping and bleeding in the stool (diverticulosis). If the diverticula become infected (a condition known as diverticulitis), antibiotics may be needed to bring the infection under control.

Fortunately, most cases of constipation can be controlled or prevented by making necessary adjustments in diet and lifestyle. It is much easier to avoid constipation or treat it in its early stages, than to try to manage the problem after complications have arisen.

Conventional Care

While an occasional bout of constipation usually can be managed at home, chronic constipation should be brought to a doctor's attention. A doctor may recommended several medical tests, such as a sigmoidoscopy, a barium enema, or a colonoscopy to rule out cancer, colitis, or an intestinal obstruction. In some cases an enlarged prostate or endometriosis can put pressure on the rectum, slowing bowel activity.

Your doctor will probably suggest you drink plenty of fluids and switch gradually to a high-fiber diet. At the same time you will be told to avoid foods that tend to be binding, such as bananas, applesauce, and white rice, which can make stools drier and harder to pass. Your doctor may also suggest you exercise to speed the movement of food through the digestive system. Try to get regular exercise, or at a minimum go for a walk after meals to stimulate the colon.

If the constipation does not respond to changes in diet and exercise, consider trying any of a number of over-the-counter laxatives or stool softeners. (In severe cases prescription laxatives may be needed.) Laxatives should be used only occasionally, to avoid creating dependence; and milk of magnesia should be avoided by people with hypertension and kidney disease, as well as by those on a low-salt diet, because it is high in sodium.

Words of Wisdom

"One problem is that many older people can't chew as well as they used to. They eat softer foods and avoid high-fiber foods, so if necessary, they need to take a fiber supplement. One way or another, we need to get our fiber."

Myrna Trowbridge, D.O.
Optimum Health Center
Valparaiso, Indiana

The Natural Approach

All of the natural remedies listed below can be used to supplement conventional medical treatment.

Herbal Medicine

Use one or more of the remedies listed below. For information on herbal medicine, see Chapter 2. Commercial preparations are also available; follow package directions.

- Aloe vera juice: This herb can heal and cleanse the digestive tract, while helping in the formation of soft stools. Take 1 tablespoon of aloe vera juice twice daily.
- Cascara sagrada *(Rhamnus purshiana):* This very pow-

erful herb contains chemicals that stimulate intestinal contractions. It is an ingredient in a number of non-prescription laxatives, as well as some prescription drugs for constipation. To prepare a decoction, boil 1 teaspoon of well-dried bark in 3 cups of water for 30 minutes. Drink one to two cups a day before bed.

- Psyllium *(Plantago psyllium):* Sometimes referred to as Mother Nature's laxative, psyllium seeds are the active ingredient in many over-the-counter laxative preparations. Take 1 to 2 rounded teaspoons after each meal in a full glass of water.
- Rhubarb *(Rheum officinale):* This herb contains laxative chemicals similar to those found in Cascara sagrada. To prepare a decoction, boil 1 to 2 teaspoons of powdered root in 1 cup of water for 10 minutes. Take 1 tablespoon at a time, up to one cup per day.

Diet and Nutrition Supplements

Use one or more of the remedies listed below. For information on nutrition supplements and good food sources of particular nutrients, see Chapter 3.

- Apple pectin: To relieve constipation, you can either eat fresh apples to enjoy their high-fiber benefits, or take 500 milligrams of apple pectin in supplement form each day.
- Fiber: Eating a diet rich in high-fiber foods—such as fruits, vegetables, whole-wheat breads, and bran—can ease constipation. Water-insoluble fibers such as cellulose (wheat bran) tend to increase stool weight by attracting and holding water. Be sure to increase your fluid intake when you increase your dietary fiber to keep stools moist and soft.
- Lactobacillus acidophilus: This supplement boosts the levels of beneficial bacteria in the intestine, which can help with digestion and relieve constipation. Take 1 teaspoon twice daily, or follow the package instructions.

- Vitamin E: This vitamin helps to heal an irritated colon. Take 400 to 800 IU a day.
- Water: Drink a minimum of eight 8-ounce glasses of water a day. Keep in mind that alcoholic and caffeinated beverages do not contribute to your daily water requirements. In fact, you should drink two glasses of water for every alcoholic or caffeinated beverage you consume.

Homeopathy

Use one homeopathic treatment at a time, based on your specific symptoms. For information on homeopathy, see Chapter 4. For dosage information, see pages 56–57. Discontinue use if the symptoms disappear.

- Alumina *(Alumina)* 6c: Use when even soft stools are difficult to pass; they may be mucus-covered or claylike. One dose every 2 hours, for up to ten doses.
- Bryonia *(Bryonia alba)* 30c: Use when the stools are large, dry, and hard. One dose every 2 hours, for up to ten doses.
- Nux *(Strychnos nux vomica)* 6c: Use when there is an urge to eliminate but little or no success in passing stools; often there is a feeling that there is more to come. One dose every 2 hours, for up to ten doses.
- Silicea *(Silicea terra)* 6c: Use when the stool passes the anal sphincter, then slips back again; stools tend to be hard and mucus-covered. One dose every 2 hours, for up to ten doses.

Acupressure

Use one or more of the acupressure points listed below. For information on acupressure, see Chapter 5. For diagrams showing the specific pressure points, see pages 88–91.

- Bladder 25: Two finger-widths on either side of the spinal column, level with the top of the hipbones.

- Conception Vessel 6: Two to three finger-widths below the belly button.
- Large Intestine 4: At the end of the crease made by the index finger and thumb when they are pressed together.
- Large Intestine 11: In the depression at the end of the elbow crease, when the elbow is slightly bent.
- Spleen 8: On the inside of the lower leg, four finger-widths below the knee, in the depression under the bone.
- Stomach 34: Three finger-widths above the kneecap, in the depression on the outer edge of the muscle.

An Ounce of Prevention

Constipation can be prevented through changes in diet and exercise habits in most cases. Be sure to drink plenty of fluids (at least eight 8-ounce glasses of water a day) and eat plenty of high-fiber foods (such as oat bran, fruits, and vegetables with skins). Regular vigorous exercise can also stimulate the bowels and relieve constipation.

Warning Signs

The telltale signs of constipation—painful bowel movements, hard and dry stools, inability to have a complete bowel movement, bloating, and gas—strike without advance warning. Constipation should be treated promptly. Not only are the symptoms unpleasant, but chronic constipation can lead to hemorrhoids, indigestion, and diverticulitis.

For More Information:

Intestinal Disease Foundation
1323 Forbes Avenue, Suite 200
Pittsburgh, PA 15219
(412) 261-5888

National Digestive Diseases Information Clearinghouse
2 Information Way
Bethesda, MD 20892-3570
(301) 654-3810

Digestive Disease National Coalition
711 2nd Street, N.E., Suite 200
Washington, DC 20002
(202) 544-7497

Dental Problems

Throughout your life your teeth require rigorous routine maintenance. If you take good care of your teeth and receive regular dental care, the vast majority of dental problems can be avoided. Despite your valiant efforts at oral hygiene, however, you may develop some dental problems. Fortunately, a number of natural remedies can be used to treat many common dental problems, including broken, cracked, or chipped teeth, tooth decay, and toothache.

Broken, Cracked, or Chipped Teeth

Like any other bone in your body, your teeth can break, crack, or chip. Sometimes all it takes to break a tooth is a firm bite down on a carrot or another hard food; other times the gradual force of grinding and clenching your teeth can damage them. And, of course, an accident or sporting mishap can lead to a less than perfect smile. In certain cases teeth with large fillings break, especially when decay has set in underneath the filling. Some breaks, cracks, and chips can be smoothed and cosmetically repaired, while others require bonding or a more extensive repair.

In general, cracks are more damaging than chips, since they reach down inside the tooth. Sometimes fine cracks defy detection, even on X rays—but you'll know the tooth is damaged, because it hurts when you chew, and it may be highly sensitive to hot and cold. Broken, cracked, or chipped teeth should be repaired as soon as possible to prevent additional damage. In some cases root canal treatment, a crown, or removal of the tooth may be necessary.

Tooth Decay

Like it or not, bacteria are always at work in the mouth, pumping out toxins that cause tooth decay. Given the chance (about twenty-four hours without brushing), the bacteria will cling to the teeth and form sticky whitish bacterial colonies known as plaque. Food debris then sticks to the plaque, allowing the plaque to grow and produce acids, which gradually erode the tooth enamel and cause cavities (or dental caries).

Cavities usually show up first as a white spot, which may later turn brown or black. (The color change depends on a number of factors, including heredity, diet, hygiene, fluoride content of the teeth, and general dental health.) To treat tooth decay, a dentist must drill out the decay and fill the tooth with amalgam, composite resins, porcelain, or gold.

Toothache

The throbbing pain of a toothache stems from exposure of the dentin, the inside of the tooth. Treatment with hot or cold packs can temporarily relieve the pain, but appropriate dental attention is needed to deal with the cause.

At some point in their lives most people experience a toothache, which can be caused by a cavity, a gum infection, a crack in the tooth, or even pressure from another dental treatment. To avoid toothaches, keep your teeth clean and seek a proper treatment when problems arise.

Conventional Care

The natural remedies recommended below are not intended to replace conventional dental care. Instead, they may be able to provide temporary relief while you seek help from a qualified dentist.

The Natural Approach

All of the natural remedies listed below can be used to supplement conventional medical treatment.

Herbal Medicine
Use one or more of the remedies listed below. For information on herbal medicine, see Chapter 2. Commercial preparations are also available; follow package directions.

For Broken, Cracked, or Chipped Tooth

- **Oil of cayenne, clove, peppermint:** To ease the pain while seeking dental attention for a broken, cracked, or chipped tooth, soak a cotton ball in any one of these oils and place it over the damaged tooth. (This also works for a toothache.)

For Toothache

- **Echinacea** *(Echinacea angustifolia):* This herb has both antibiotic and anti-inflammatory properties. To prepare a tea, add 1 heaping teaspoon of herb to a cup of boiling water, and steep for 5 minutes; strain, and drink up to three cups a day.

- Goldenseal *(Hydrastis canadensis):* This herb also has antibiotic and anti-inflammatory properties. To prepare a tea, add 1 heaping teaspoon of herb to 1 cup of boiling water and steep for 5 minutes; strain, and drink up to three cups a day.
- Marjoram *(Origanum majorana):* To soothe the pain of a toothache, as well as to promote restful sleep, try marjoram tea. Use 1 heaping teaspoon of dried herb per cup of boiling water. Steep for 5 minutes, strain, and drink two or three cups a day.
- Saltwater rinse: A warm saltwater rinse or a solution of 1 cup warm saltwater mixed with 1 tablespoon of aloe vera gel may reduce gum irritation and tooth pain. To prepare the saltwater mixture, stir 1 teaspoon of table salt into 1 cup of warm water.

Diet and Nutrition Supplements

Use one or more of the remedies listed below. For information on nutrition supplements and good food sources of particular nutrients, see Chapter 3.

For Overall Dental Health

- **Calcium:** Healthy teeth and bones require sufficient calcium. Take up to 1,500 milligrams a day.
- Magnesium: Calcium and magnesium work together to promote healthy teeth and bones. Take up to 750 milligrams a day, along with the calcium.
- Zinc: This mineral promotes immune function and tissue healing. Take up to 50 milligrams a day.

Homeopathy

Use one homeopathic treatment at a time, based on your specific symptoms. For information on homeopathy, see Chapter 4. For dosage information, see pages 56–57. Discontinue use if the symptoms disappear.

For Broken, Cracked, or Chipped Teeth

- **Chamomilla** *(Chamomilla vulgaris)* 30x: Use when pain from a broken, cracked, or chipped tooth worsens when exposed to heat. One dose every hour, for up to six hours.
- Hypericum *(Hypericum perforatum)* 30x: Use after dental treatment for a broken, cracked, or chipped tooth to prevent long-lasting nerve damage. One dose three times a day, for one week.

For Tooth Decay

- **Kreosotum** *(Kreosotum)* 6c: Use when the decayed teeth have turned black. One dose twice a day, for three weeks.
- Mercurius *(Mercurius solubilis hahnemanni)* 6c: Use when decayed teeth are decayed and loose. One dose twice a day, for three weeks.

For Toothache

- **Arnica** *(Arnica montana)* 30x: Use to relieve toothache pain that is worse at night. One dose every 15 minutes, as needed. (Also use for pain after dental treatment; one dose hourly for up to ten doses.)
- Belladonna *(Atropa belladonna)* 30c: Use when a toothache includes a throbbing pain, shooting from the ear. The gums and cheeks may be swollen and hot (signs of infection). One dose every 5 minutes, for up to ten doses.
- Chamomilla *(Chamomilla vulgaris)* 30x: Use for toothache that becomes worse when exposed to heat. One dose hourly, as needed.
- Coffea *(Coffea cruda)* 6c: Use when sharp, shooting pain accompanies an aching tooth; pain is relieved by ice water. One dose every 5 minutes, for up to ten doses.

Acupressure

Use one or more of the acupressure points listed below. For information on acupressure, see Chapter 5. For diagrams showing the specific pressure points, see pages 88–91.

For Overall Dental Health

- **Gallbladder 2:** Behind the jawbone and in front of the earlobe, in the depression formed when the mouth is open.
- Stomach 3: Along the cheekbone, in line with the pupil of the eye, and level with the outside edge of the nostril.
- Stomach 4: Just below Stomach 3, at the corner of the mouth. Also stimulates salivation.
- Triple Warmer 21: In the slight hollow located just in front of the notch at the top of the ear. Try opening your mouth to pinpoint the location of the depression.

For Toothache

- **Kidney 3:** Inside the ankle, in the depression halfway between the anklebone and the back of the ankle.
- Large Intestine 4: In the webbing between the thumb and index finger, located at the end of the crease formed when the thumb and index finger are pressed together.
- Small Intestine 19: In the depression directly in front of the ear opening; the depression becomes deeper when the mouth is opened.
- Stomach 7: On the side of the cheek, in the hollow along the cheekbone and in front of the earlobe.

An Ounce of Prevention

Most dental problems can be avoided by brushing and flossing your teeth properly to clean them and remove plaque.

Most dentists recommend brushing after every meal, but they realize that brushing morning and night are all most people are willing to do. However, a complete job once a day is better than two or three quick and superficial brushings. Use fluoride toothpaste to further protect the teeth.

To avoid long-term problems, you should visit the dentist for a checkup and professional cleaning twice a year. Regular cleanings not only prevent tooth decay and toothache, they can also slow or prevent periodontal disease (see page 371). And if you engage in athletics or other high-impact activities, be sure to wear a mouth guard to minimize the risk of chipped or broken teeth.

Warning Signs

If you get regular checkups, you'll probably hear about your problems right from the dentist's mouth. If you are less fortunate and a problem progresses to the point where it becomes painful, a throbbing toothache will let you know that something has gone wrong.

While you probably won't be able to see any dental caries (cavities), you may be able to feel the trouble spots where plaque has built up. Run your tongue across the surface of your teeth. Your teeth should feel smooth, not gritty or coated with fuzz. If you can see or feel plaque or tartar, take special care to brush and floss the area thoroughly.

For More Information:

American Dental Association
211 East Chicago Avenue
Chicago, IL 60611
(312) 440-2500

American Society for Geriatric Dentistry
211 East Chicago Avenue, Suite 948
Chicago, IL 60611
(312) 440-2661

National Dental Association
5506 Connecticut Avenue, N.W., Suite 24
Washington, DC 20015
(202) 244-7555

Holistic Dental Association
P.O. Box 5007
Durango, CO 81301
(970) 259-1091

Depression

At some point in their lives, most people experience depression. Though many people confuse the two, depression isn't the same thing as sadness. While we all feel sadness in response to certain situations—the death of a loved one, the loss of a job, a divorce, or some other disappointment—depression is characterized by ongoing feelings of worthlessness, pessimism, sadness, and lack of interest in life. With clinical depression these feelings linger for weeks or months and ultimately become incapacitating.

Depression can be either a short-term, minor problem or a lifelong, life-threatening illness. In fact, more than four out of five people who commit suicide are depressed, and the suicide rate among older people is three to four times higher than the rate for the general population.

According to the National Institute of Mental Health, an estimated 10 to 15 percent of older Americans experience depression severe enough to require treatment. Some people inherit a tendency to develop depression due to their brain chemistry. Other times the illness is brought-on by physical conditions, such as stroke, hepatitis, chronic fatigue syndrome, chronic stress, thyroid disease, menopause, alcoholism, or drug abuse—or even by the lack of natural light during the darker winter months. Some drugs, including over-the-counter antihistamines as well as many others, can cause depression too.

Whatever the cause, most cases of depression involve an imbalance of neurotransmitters, or chemical messengers in the brain. While depression was once considered a shameful psychiatric condition, most experts now recognize that it usually has both physical and psychological triggers. It is an organic illness involving physical, biochemical changes in the body, so without help the person cannot "snap out of it," no matter how hard they try. While counseling and professional care can be crucial in recovery, a number of natural remedies may also prove useful.

Conventional Care

When it comes to dealing with depression, most mental health professionals rely on three types of treatment—counseling (psychotherapy or "talk therapy"), medication (drug therapy), and electroconvulsive therapy (ECT or "shock therapy"). These techniques can be used alone or in combination. Because depression can be caused by a wide variety of factors working together, a combination approach is often most successful.

Words of Wisdom

"You cannot separate the mind and the body: Anything you do to enhance your physical health will enhance your mental health and help to relieve depression. Take the antioxidants to support your body. Make friends and maintain relationships that provide social support. And don't forget that the later years can be very rich and rewarding. People worry about getting older and going over the hill, but they forget: Once you're over the hill, you get to coast."

Henry Edward Altenberg, M.D.
Co-director, Spruce Creek Holistic Center
Rochester, New Hampshire
Attending Geriatric Psychiatrist
Frisbee Memorial Hospital
Kittery, Maine

The Natural Approach

All of the natural remedies listed below can be used to supplement conventional medical treatment.

Herbal Medicine

Use one or more of the remedies listed below. For information on herbal medicine, see Chapter 2. Commercial preparations are also available; follow package directions.

- Basil *(Ocimum basilicum):* This herb has antidepressant properties, and some believe it to be spiritually uplifting. Eat fresh basil leaves; add 5 drops of essential oil of basil to bathwater.
- Oats *(Avena sativa):* Run-of-the-mill oats and oatmeal have antidepressant and mood-elevating properties. Eat oatmeal cereal, or take a commercially prepared oat extract.
- St. John's wort *(Hypericum perforatum):* This herb has long been used as a mood enhancer and antidepressant. It contains a chemical (hypericin) that blocks the action of monoamine oxidase (MAO) in the body. (MAO inhibitors are a common class of prescription antidepressant drugs.) For an infusion, use 1 to 2 teaspoons of dried herb per cup of boiling water. Steep 10 to 15 minutes, strain, and drink up to three cups a day. *Note:* While taking the herb, do not take amphet-

amines, narcotics, diet pills, asthma inhalants, decongestants, or cold or hay fever medication.

Diet and Nutrition Supplements

Use one or more of the remedies listed below. For information on nutrition supplements and good food sources of particular nutrients, see Chapter 3.

- Calcium and magnesium: Studies have shown that people who experience depression often have low levels of calcium and magnesium. Take up to 1,500 milligrams of calcium and 750 milligrams of magnesium a day.
- Vitamin C: This vitamin is necessary for the synthesis of neurotransmitters in the brain. Take up to 3,000 milligrams a day, in divided doses.

Homeopathy

Use one homeopathic treatment at a time, based on your specific symptoms. For information on homeopathy, see Chapter 4. For dosage information, see pages 56–57. Discontinue use if the symptoms disappear.

- Aurum *(Aurum metallicum)* 6c: Use when suicidal feelings and self-loathing accompany depression. One dose three times a day, for two weeks. *Note:* If someone feels suicidal, seek professional help or call a suicide hotline in addition to using natural remedies.
- Ignatia *(Ignatia amara)* 6c: Use when depression follows a heartbreak or deep grief and is accompanied by mood swings; behavior may be inappropriate for a given situation. One dose three times a day, for up to two weeks.
- Nux *(Strychnos nux vomica)* 6c: Use when depression is accompanied by irritability. One dose three times a day, for two weeks.
- Pulsatilla *(Pulsatilla nigricans)* 6c: Use when tearfulness and self-pity accompany depression. One dose three times a day, for up to two weeks.

Acupressure

Use one or more of the acupressure points listed below. For information on acupressure, see Chapter 5. For diagrams showing the specific pressure points, see pages 88–91.

- Bladder 10: Just inside the hairline on the nape of the neck, a half-inch out on either side of the spine, in the depression on the side of the large neck muscles.
- Conception Vessel 12: Along the center of the abdomen, halfway between the navel and the edge of the breastbone.
- Governing Vessel 26: Halfway up the groove below the nose. *Note:* Avoid using this pressure point if you have high blood pressure.
- Liver 3: On the top of the foot, in the web between the first and second toes.

An Ounce of Prevention

Sadness is part of life, but clinical depression doesn't have to be. Debilitating depression should be treated by a mental health professional. But you may be able to prevent some types of depression—as well as generally elevate your mood—by getting regular exercise and rest and by sharing your feelings with someone you trust. Be aware that depression and sadness can also be a side effect of many medications, including over-the-counter antihistamines. If you suspect your mood changes are drug induced, talk to your doctor.

Warning Signs

It can be difficult to tell the difference between clinical depression and common sadness. But there are certain warning signs:

- Changes in sleep—to either insomnia or sleepiness
- Changes in weight and eating habits: either weight gain or weight loss
- Loss of sexual desire or libido
- Chronic fatigue or tiredness
- Low self-esteem or self-worth
- Loss of productivity at work, home, or school
- Inability to concentrate or think clearly
- Withdrawal or isolation
- Loss of interest in activities that were once enjoyable
- Anger or irritability
- Trouble accepting praise or affirmation
- Feeling slow, every activity takes supreme effort
- Apprehension about the future
- Frequent weeping or sobbing
- Thoughts of suicide or death

These are all warnings signs and diagnostic criteria for depression. If you or a loved one experiences three or more of them for two weeks or longer, contact a doctor or mental health professional for help. Don't try to treat serious depression by yourself. And if you or someone you're concerned about feels suicidal, immediately seek help from a specialist or a twenty-four-hour hotline; look in the phone book under "Suicide Prevention."

For More Information:

Depressives Anonymous: Recovering from Depression
329 East 62nd Street
New York, NY 10021
(212) 689-2600

Depression and Related Affective Disorders Association
Johns Hopkins Hospital
600 North Wolfe Street
Baltimore, MD 21287
(410) 955-4647

Depression Awareness, Recognition, and Treatment (D/ART)
(800) 421-4211

Foundation for Depression and Manic Depression
24 East 81st Street, Suite 2B
New York, NY 10028
(212) 772-3400

National Mental Health Association
1021 Prince Street
Alexandria, VA 22314
(703) 684-7722
(800) 243-2525

National Depressive and Manic Depressive Association
730 North Franklin Street, Suite 501
Chicago, IL 60610
(312) 642-0049
(800) 826-3632

National Foundation for Depressive Illness
P.O. Box 2257
New York, NY 10116
(212) 268-4260

Diabetes

For diabetics, life is a balancing act. They must carefully watch their blood-sugar levels: If the levels rise too high and stay there for too long, they risk damage to the nerves and blood vessels, which can cause a number of health problems, including blindness, infection, kidney problems, stroke, and heart disease. But if blood-sugar levels drop too low—even for a few minutes—they can become confused and even lose consciousness.

Normally the pancreas regulates this delicate balance of sugar in the bloodstream. But the fourteen million Americans with diabetes mellitus cannot properly convert food (especially sugar) into energy, either because their bodies do not produce enough insulin (a hormone produced in the pancreas to regulate blood-sugar levels) or because their bodies don't properly use the insulin they do produce. Instead, diabetics must monitor their blood-sugar levels, adjusting their diet and exercise—or their oral medications and insulin injections—to meet these changing conditions.

There are two basic types of diabetes: the more severe form, known as Type I, insulin-dependent, or juvenile diabetes (about 15 percent of cases); and Type II, noninsulin-dependent, or adult-onset diabetes (about 85 percent of cases).

- Type I diabetes usually strikes sometime between the onset of puberty and age 30. It is caused by damage to the insulin-producing cells in the pancreas. For some reason it affects males more often than females.
- Type II diabetes usually occurs in middle-aged and older people, especially those who are overweight. Losing as little as ten or fifteen pounds helps control Type II diabetes in most cases. With Type II diabetes the pancreas produces insulin, but the sugar remains in the bloodstream. This more subtle version of the disease often goes undetected, until complications arise. Ultimately, up to 60 percent of Type II diabetics need supplemental insulin.

Both Type I and Type II diabetes seem to have a genetic component as well. Other possible causes include an immune response, following a viral infection, that destroys the cells in the pancreas. Diabetes can also follow other diseases, such as thyroid disorders, inflammation of the pancreas, or problems with the pituitary gland. In addition, about 5 percent of women develop diabetes when pregnant, though the symptoms usually disappear after the baby is born.

Conventional Care

The standard treatment for diabetes focuses on controlling blood-sugar levels, relieving symptoms, and preventing complications associated with the disease. To confirm the diagnosis, a doctor administers a glucose-tolerance test, which measures the body's reaction to sugar.

Many cases of diabetes can be controlled through weight loss, diet, and regular exercise. Medication and insulin injections may be needed in some cases to lower blood-sugar levels.

Diabetics must also take steps to protect their feet, teeth, and gums. Nerve damage associated with the disease can reduce sensation in the feet, leaving them susceptible to injuries and infections, which don't heal well due to blood vessel damage. Simple cuts and scrapes can easily become gangrenous. (See page 255 for information on diabetic feet.) In addition, diabetics tend to develop more tooth and gum infections.

Words of Wisdom

"Herbs can help someone with adult-onset diabetes get off insulin, and they can help someone with juvenile-onset diabetes avoid complications associated with the disease. I know because I am a diabetic. I developed diabetes when I was 10, and 36 years later my eyes, my kidneys, my lungs, my liver all are perfect. Without insulin, I would have died in 1966. The insulin saved my life, but the herbal remedies have made my life worth living."

Alan Tillotson, M.A.
Member of the American Herbalists Guild
Director, Chrysalis Natural Medicine Clinic
Wilmington, Delaware

The Natural Approach

All of the natural remedies listed below can be used to supplement conventional medical treatment.

Herbal Medicine

Use one or more of the remedies listed below. For more information on herbal medicine, see Chapter 2. Commercial preparations are also available; follow package directions.

- Fenugreek *(Trigonella foenum-gracecum):* Studies have shown that this herb can reduce urine sugar levels by 50 percent. For a decoction, gently boil 2 teaspoons of bruised seeds per cup of water; simmer 10 minutes, strain, and drink up to three cups a day.
- Garlic *(Allium sativum):* This herb helps lower blood-sugar levels. Eat 3 to 6 cloves of garlic a day, or use a commercially prepared product.
- Ginseng *(Panax quinquefolius):* This herb helps to reduce blood-sugar levels. Commercial products are available at health food stores.
- Sage *(Salvia officinalis):* Studies show that sage lowers blood-sugar levels when consumed on an empty stomach. For an infusion, use 1 to 2 teaspoons of dried leaves per cup of boiling water; steep for 10 minutes. Drink up to three cups a day.

Diet and Nutrition Supplements

Use one or more of the remedies listed below. For information on nutrition supplements and good food sources of particular nutrients, see Chapter 3.

- Chromium: Studies have found that people with adult-onset diabetes can lower their insulin requirements by taking chromium supplements. Chromium makes insulin about ten times more efficient at processing sugar, so less insulin is needed to do the job.

Unfortunately, levels of chromium in the body tend to decrease with age. Under a doctor's supervision, take 200 micrograms of chromium a day. (A doctor should monitor the impact of chromium supplementation on the body, since large fluctuations in blood-glucose levels should be avoided.)

- Fiber: Soluble fiber has been shown to help keep blood sugar under control. To help control glucose levels, eat a diet rich in beans and other foods high in soluble fiber. They type of bean doesn't matter, so enjoy red, white, and navy beans; lentils, garbanzos, and pinto beans. Soluble fiber supplements are also available from health food stores.
- Magnesium: Many diabetics have a deficiency in magnesium; supplements (even at low doses) tend to minimize complications related to the disease. Take 300 milligrams of magnesium chloride a day.
- Vitamin E: This vitamin helps the body maintain normal glucose or blood-sugar levels. Take 400 to 800 IU a day.

Homeopathy

Use one homeopathic treatment at a time, based on your specific symptoms. For information on homeopathy, see Chapter 2. For dosage information, see pages 56–57. Discontinue use if the symptoms disappear.

- Argentum nit. *(Argentum nitricum)* 6c: Use when swollen ankles accompany other diabetic symptoms. One dose four times a day, for up to two weeks.
- Phosphoric ac. *(Phosphoricum acidum)* 6c: Use when nervous exhaustion accompanies other diabetic symptoms. One dose four times a day, for up to two weeks.
- Silicea *(Silicea terra)* 6c: Use when sweaty feet and fatigue accompany other diabetic symptoms. One dose four times a day, for up to two weeks.

An Ounce of Prevention

While not all cases of diabetes can be prevented, many can. Maintain a healthy weight (most diabetics weigh 30 to 60 pounds more than they should); eat a low-fat, high-fiber diet; and of course, exercise regularly. Studies have shown that vigorous exercise can lower the risk of developing Type II diabetes by one-third. In fact, many experts consider exercise the most effective way to prevent noninsulin-dependent diabetes. (For more information on exercise, see Chapter 6.)

Warning Signs

Diabetes can be difficult to detect. In fact, only about half of all diabetics know they have the disease. The symptoms of Type I diabetes—excessive thirst, frequent urination, dry mouth, blurred vision, and frequent infections—often develop rapidly. The signs of Type II diabetes—thirst, drowsiness, obesity, fatigue, tingling or numbness in the feet, blurred vision, and itching—often go unrecognized for years before being properly diagnosed.

For More Information:

American Diabetes Association
National Center
P.O. Box 25757
1660 Duke Street
Alexandria, VA 22314
(703) 549-1500

Diabetes Research Institute Foundation
3440 Hollywood Boulevard, Suite 100
Hollywood, FL 33021
(305) 964-4040

International Diabetes Center
3800 Park Nicollet Boulevard
Minneapolis, MN 55416
(612) 927-3393

Joslin Diabetes Center
One Joslin Place
Boston, MA 02215
(617) 732-2415

Foot Problems

Feet get no respect. We spend years cramming our toes into pointy-toed pumps, exposing our feet to fungus-covered floors in wet locker rooms, and suffocating our soles in tight nylon hosiery. Then after decades of abusing our dogs, we gripe when they bark back.

Your feet deserve better. In fact, each foot is a remarkable feat of biological engineering. Its 28 bones, 33 joints, and complex web of more than a hundred tendons, muscles, and ligaments allow us to walk, run, skip, dance, and tiptoe. During the average day our feet support a cumulative force equal to several hundred tons.

As a result, our feet can develop a wide range of problems, from calluses and corns to blisters and bunions and burning soles. In addition, as a normal part of the aging process, we lose connective-tissue elasticity, which eventually leads to the loss of the heel and forefoot shock-absorbing pads. Heel pain is quite common as we age, mainly because of the loss of this fatty-cell cushioning.

As we grow older, our foot structure also changes: The forefoot widens, flattens, and may even lengthen. Shoe-fitting problems become more significant since people often fail to realize (or stubbornly refuse to admit) that their feet have grown larger. The painful result: People jam their feet into ill-fitting shoes.

Painful feet can force the entire body out of alignment. One problem can lead to another, as foot troubles can force an unnatural gait, which puts stress on the knees and hips and can contribute to osteoarthritis. But many foot problems can be avoided by wearing appropriate shoes and by using natural remedies to address minor problems before they become severe.

Conventional Care

Treatments for various foot conditions vary, depending on the cause of the problem.

The Natural Approach

All of the natural remedies listed below can be used to supplement conventional medical treatment.

Herbal Medicine

Use one or more of the remedies listed below. For information on herbal medicine, see Chapter 2. Commercial preparations are also available; follow package directions.

Burning Feet

- **Eucalyptus** *(Eucalyptus globulus)* **and rosemary** *(Rosmarinus officinalis):* To relieve burning feet, soak your feet for 5 minutes in a shallow tub of hot water containing 6 drops of eucalyptus oil and 6 drops of rosemary oil. Let the oils soothe and relax you. The oils are available in health food stores.

* Red pepper *(Capsicum annuum):* Extracts of this hot pepper help to relieve the severe ankle and foot pain known as burning-foot syndrome, a common complaint of diabetics. For external application to help treat pain, mix 1/4 to 1/2 teaspoon of pepper per cup of warm vegetable oil, and rub into the affected area.

Muscle Cramps

* **Mexican wild yam** *(Dioscorea villosa):* This herb relaxes the muscles and the peripheral blood vessels, making it a good treatment for muscle spasms. Commercial preparations are available; follow package directions.

Warts

* **Tea tree oil** *(Melaleuca alternifolia):* This powerful antibiotic is useful for fungal, bacterial, and viral infections. Apply 2 or 3 drops of essential oil directly on the wart for as long as necessary until the wart disappears.

Homeopathy

Use one homeopathic treatment at a time, based on your specific symptoms. For information on homeopathy, see Chapter 5. For dosage information, see pages 56–57. Discontinue use if the symptoms disappear.

* Apis *(Apis mellifica)* 30c: Use when your feet feel burning, stiff, and swollen. One dose every 4 hours, for up to three doses.
* Arnica *(Arnica montana)* 30c: Use when your feet ache after too much walking or standing. One dose every 4 hours, for up to three doses.
* Muriatic ac. *(Muriaticum acidum)* 30c: Use when the soles of your feet hurt and you feel tightness in your

Achilles tendons. One dose every 4 hours, for up to three doses.

- Nitric ac. *(Nitricum acidum)* 30c: Use when the soles of your feet feel as if you're walking on pins and needles. One dose every 4 hours, for up to three doses.

Acupressure

Use one or more of the acupressure points listed below. For information on acupressure, see Chapter 5. For diagrams showing the specific pressure points, see pages 88–91. These points all relieve pain and swelling in the feet, heels, and ankles.

- Bladder 60: In the depression behind the anklebone, on the outside edge of the ankle.
- Bladder 62: In the hollow directly below the outer anklebone; this point is one-third the distance from the outer anklebone to the bottom of the heel.
- Kidney 1: On the sole of the foot, in the depression just below the ball of the foot.

An Ounce of Prevention

You can avoid a lot of foot problems by buying only comfortable shoes that fit properly. That means living without high-fashion shoes with pointed toes and stiletto heels and opting instead for roomy shoes that are actually shaped like feet. Follow these shoe-fitting tips:

- When buying shoes, shop in the late afternoon or evening, since your feet swell during the day.
- Make sure there's between 3/8 and 1/2 inch of space between the tip of your longest toe and the end of the shoe. You should have plenty of room to wiggle your toes and allow air to circulate. When it comes to width, make sure the ball of your foot isn't squeezed uncomfortably. And of course, always try on both shoes, since few people have feet of identical size.

- No matter how much you like them, never buy shoes expecting that they will stretch to fit. If they're tight in the store, they'll be tight when you get home.
- Look for shoes made of leather, canvas, or other materials that allow your feet to breathe. Fake leather (as well as real leather with a waterproof coating) can trap perspiration inside, creating a warm, moist breeding ground for odor-causing bacteria and fungi.
- Take care to keep your feet clean and dry. If your feet sweat a lot, use cornstarch powder between your toes, wear cotton socks, and change them often.

Warning Signs

Pain is the body's warning sign that something is rubbing your feet the wrong way. Heed your body's warning, and remove your shoes before a minor irritation becomes a major problems.

For More Information:

American Association of Podiatric Physicians and Surgeons
1328 Southern Avenue, S.E., Suite 200
Washington, DC 20032
(202) 562-2777

American College of Foot and Ankle Surgeons
515 Busse Highway
Park Ridge, IL 60068
(708) 292-2237

American Podiatric Medical Association
9312 Old Georgetown Road
Bethesda, MD 20814
(301) 571-9200

Taking Care of Diabetic Feet

While most people suffer from painful feet every once in a while, diabetics face special foot care problems. Many diabetics develop a condition known as neuropathy, or nerve damage to the feet and legs, which results in burning, pain, and numbness. More important, due to the loss of feeling, minor injuries, blisters, and sores often go undetected until they become infected. In severe cases these problems can lead to gangrene and even amputation.

But there are steps that you can take to avoid problems:

- **Examine your feet daily.** As part of your daily routine, schedule time to give your feet a thorough check to make sure you haven't developed a sore, blister, cut, scrape, or other problem that could become more serious. If you find it difficult to bend and reach your feet, ask someone else to assist you in your foot check.

- **Keep your feet clean.** The cleaner your feet, the lower the risk of infection. Wash them thoroughly every day, and dry them carefully to reduce the formation of bacteria.

- **Treat your feet with TLC.** Diabetic feet need tender loving care, especially when they develop corns and calluses. While you might be tempted to treat these relatively minor foot care problems at home, seek professional help from a podiatrist or general practitioner. Using a razor, caustic agents, or even a pumice stone can cause serious problems.

- **Don't let minor irritations become major problems.** Immediately tend to any cut, scape, blister, burn, or injury by washing it thoroughly with soap and water and covering it with a protective sterile dressing to minimize the risk of infection.

- **Never go barefoot.** The best way to protect your feet from injury is to wear shoes—all the time.

- **Make sure the shoe fits.** It is especially difficult for diabetics with neuropathy to choose shoes that fit since they cannot feel the pain associated with a snug fit or friction. Take special care when shopping for shoes to select those that are wide enough, have plenty of room in the toe box, and don't slip at the heel.

Gallstones and Gallbladder Disease

Gallstones are unpredictable: They can be smaller than a pea or larger than an egg. They can sit quietly and not cause any trouble or they can block the bile duct or become inflamed, resulting in severe pain in the upper right abdomen, often accompanied by fever, nausea, and vomiting.

Gallbladder disease is serious business. Untreated, gallbladder inflammation (also called *cholecystitis*) can be life threatening. If the bile duct is blocked by a gallstone, bile can back up in the system, causing the skin and whites of the eyes to turn yellow with jaundice and the urine to turn dark brown.

These complications arise from problems with the concentration of bile, the yellowish substance the body uses to digest fats. The liver produces bile (which consists of cholesterol, bile salts, and lecithin, among other substances),

256

and any surplus is stored in the gallbladder, a small organ nestled under the liver. If the bile in the gallbladder becomes too concentrated, the cholesterol can crystalize, forming gallstones. While 80 percent of all gallstones are composed primarily of cholesterol, they can also be formed of pure bile or mixtures of bile, cholesterol, and calcium.

Women tend to develop gallbladder disease more often than men; as many as one out of four women over age 55 has gallstones. Extra pounds put you at extra risk of developing gallstones; people more than 20 percent overweight double their risk of developing gallbladder disease. Other risk factors include eating a high-fat and high-sugar diet, rapid weight loss, lack of exercise, diabetes, hypertension, and estrogen replacement therapy (the estrogen increases the cholesterol levels in the bile). Native Americans are also at high risk.

While chronic gallbladder disease often results in the surgical removal of the gallbladder (a procedure known as a cholecystectomy), many people can control the disease by making dietary changes and using nutritional supplements and other natural remedies.

Conventional Care

Like many medical conditions, gallstones are easier to prevent than to cure. To assist in the diagnosis, a physician may order a cholecystogram, a type of gallbladder X ray, an ultrasound scan, or a CAT scan. These diagnostic tests help reveal the condition of the gallbladder so that a course of treatment can be established. Once gallbladder disease is diagnosed, your doctor will recommend changes in diet to control the irritation and to minimize the risk of new stones forming.

Certain types of small gallstones may dissolve in response to prescription drugs. But in most chronic or severe cases, surgery is necessary to remove the gallstones and sometimes the entire gallbladder. (Gallbladder surgery is the fifth most common surgical procedure in the United States.) Surgical options also include laser surgery and a technique in which the gallbladder is infused with a strong chemical solution that dissolves the cholesterol.

In addition, your doctor will probably recommend that you drink at least eight 8-ounce glasses of water a day. The water helps the body produce the right concentration of bile, which can help prevent the formation of gallstones.

Many doctors recommend that you eat a number of small meals throughout the day—starting with breakfast. Prolonged periods of fasting can cause the bile to sit in the gallbladder too long, increasing the risk of developing new gallstones.

The Natural Approach

All of the natural remedies listed below can be used to supplement conventional medical treatment.

Herbal Medicine

Use one or more of the remedies listed below. For information on herbal medicine, see Chapter 2. Commercial preparations are also available; follow package directions.

- Barberry *(Berberis vulgaris):* This herb encourages the flow of bile and helps with liver congestion. (It also has a laxative effect.) For a decoction, add 1 teaspoon of dried herb to a cup of boiling water and simmer for 15 minutes, then strain and drink. Commercially prepared tinctures are available; follow package directions.
- Dandelion *(Taraxacum officinale):* This herb (or weed, depending on your point of view) enhances liver and gallbladder function. Dandelion is rich in lecithin, which helps control cholesterol. Eat fresh dandelion in salads, or use commercially available capsules, following package directions.

- Fringe tree *(Chionanthus virginicus):* This herb helps to stimulate liver function and the flow of bile. Commercially prepared tinctures are available; follow package directions.
- Turmeric *(Curcuma longa):* Studies performed in Germany and India show that this spice (an ingredient in curry) may help to prevent gallstones by enhancing the action of the liver and gallbladder. Use it in cooking, or use commercially available products, following package directions.

Diet and Nutrition Supplements

Use one or more of the remedies listed below. For information on nutrition supplements and good food sources of particular nutrients, see Chapter 3.

- Lecithin: Supplements of lecithin can help control cholesterol buildup and prevent gallstones. Lecithin is sold in granule and capsule form at natural food stores. Follow package directions.
- Low-fat diet: Stick to a low-fat diet. Too much fat in the diet can cause the liver to overproduce bile, which in turn can cause gallstones.
- Vitamin C: A deficiency in vitamin C has been linked to the formation of gallstones. Take up to 3,000 milligrams a day.

Homeopathy

Use one homeopathic treatment at a time, based on your specific symptoms. For information on homeopathy, see Chapter 4. For dosage information, see pages 56–57. Discontinue use if the symptoms disappear.

- Berberis *(Berberis vulgaris)* 6c: Use when gallstones have been diagnosed. One dose four times a day, for up to two weeks.
- China *(China officinalis)* 6c: Use if gallstones are pres-

ent and berberis has proven ineffective. One dose four times a day, for up to two weeks.

Acupressure
For information on acupressure, see Chapter 5. For diagrams showing this pressure point, see pages 88–91.

- Gallbladder 34: On the outside of the leg, in the hollow just beneath the meeting point of the two leg bones, one thumb-width above and two finger-widths to the outside of Stomach 36.

An Ounce of Prevention

To prevent gallstones and gallbladder disease, you should treat your body with the dietary respect it deserves. Eat a diet high in fiber and low in fats, sugars, and cholesterol. Exercise regularly. Avoid smoking or spending time around people who do. Maintain your ideal weight, and avoid crash diets and rapid weight-loss programs, which can cause gallstones. (For more information on weight loss, see Chapter 8.)

Warning Signs

Most people with gallstones and gallbladder disease experience the classic symptoms of digestive distress—bloating, gas, and nausea—especially after eating a fatty meal. However, between one-third and one-half of all people with gallstones actually have no pains or warning symptoms—until they suffer from the excruciating pain, on the right side of the abdomen or between the shoulder blades, associated with passing a gallstone.

For more information:

National Digestive Disease Information Clearinghouse
2 Information Way
Bethesda, MD 20892-3570
(301) 654-3810

Gout

Sometimes stereotypes have a grain of truth in them. So it is with gout. This condition earned a reputation as "the rich man's disease" because it tended to afflict overweight, wealthy men who consumed a diet high in red meat and wine. This description may not be too far from the mark, since eating meat and drinking alcohol can contribute to the disease.

Gout is a relatively common type of arthritis caused by the buildup of uric acid, a by-product of the metabolism of purines, which are made by the body and consumed in foods. During a "gout attack," the uric acid forms tiny crystals of sodium urate, which collect in a joint (often the big toe), causing inflammation and severe pain. The red-meat-and-wine stereotype makes sense when you consider that meats (especially organ meats) contain high levels of purines, and alcohol (including wine) interferes with the ability of the kidneys to excrete uric acids.

Gout affects about one million Americans, mostly men over age 40.

Gout doesn't appear overnight. In some cases, it may take years or even decades for uric acid crystals to build up before an attack. Gout can strike the heel, ankle, or instep, but more than half the time the first attack afflicts the first joint of the big toe. (The big toe may be the most frequent target because uric acid crystallizes more easily at lower temperatures, and the body temperature is somewhat lower in the toes and lower extremities than at the body's core.) Often the acute pain strikes in the middle of the night, especially after overindulging in food and alcohol. Fever and chills may accompany the pain.

About half of all gout sufferers have a second attack within one year, and three-fourths will have a recurrence within four to five years. But chronic gout is rare and unnecessary, since the condition can be controlled by diet and drug therapy designed to lower uric acid levels. Some people develop elevated uric acid levels and gout as a side effect of another disorder, such as kidney disease, which can inhibit uric acid excretion. Low-dose aspirin therapy and some diuretic high-blood-pressure treatments can also cause gout.

Conventional Care

Doctors can confirm the diagnosis of gout by testing the uric acid levels in the blood, or by withdrawing a sample of joint fluid to look for evidence of crystals. Most cases of gout can be managed by diet alone, but a number of drugs may also prove useful in managing gout attacks. Antigout drugs include colchicine (which lowers the acidity of the joints, stopping the inflammation and dissolving the uric acid crystals), allopurinol (used when the body produces too much uric acid), and sulfinpyrazone (used when the body excretes too little uric acid).

The Natural Approach

All of the natural remedies listed below can be used to supplement conventional medical treatment.

Herbal Medicine

Use one or more of the remedies listed below. For more information on herbal medicine, see Chapter 2. Commercial preparations are also available; follow package directions.

- Devil's claw *(Harpagophytum porcumbens):* This herb has both anti-inflammatory and analgesic effects; it contains a chemical, harpagoside, which reduces joint inflammation. It also has been shown to lower uric acid levels. For an infusion, add 1 to 2 teaspoons of dried herb to 1 cup of boiling water. Steep for 15 minutes. Strain, and drink up to two cups a day.
- Nettle *(Urtica dioica):* The external use of nettle can help treat gout pain. Though it may sound masochistic, urtication (flailing yourself with the stinging plant) helps relieve gout pain. The fresh plant can also be placed in a juicer to generate nettle juice, which can be applied topically to the affected joint.

Diet and Nutrition Supplements

Use one or more of the recommendations listed below. For information on nutrition supplements and good food sources of particular nutrients, see Chapter 3.

- Flavonoids: Cherries, blueberries, and other dark red or blue berries contain high levels of flavonoid compounds called anthocyanidins and proanthocyanidins. Eating a half-pound of these berries a day helps lower uric acid levels.
- Fluids: Drinking lots of fluids, especially water, dilutes the urine and encourages the body to excrete excess uric acid.

Foods to Avoid

When it comes to preventing and treating gout, what you don't eat is as important as—or more important than—what you do eat. Avoid the following foods:

- **Alcohol:** Alcohol increases levels of gout-causing uric acid in the bloodstream by impairing the kidney's ability to excrete the substance. As a result, drinking alcohol can trigger a gout attack.
- **Carbohydrates and saturated fats:** Minimize your intake of refined carbohydrates (which increase the production of uric acid in the blood) and saturated fats (which decrease the secretion of uric acid in the blood).
- **Purines:** Cutting purine-containing foods from your diet is one of the best ways to control outbreaks of gout. That means eliminating anchovies, brewer's and baker's yeast, herring, mackerel, organ meat, sardines, and shellfish.
- **Vitamin C:** Megadoses of vitamin C can actually increase levels of uric acid in the blood. Skip the vitamin C supplements if you have gout.

Homeopathy

Use one homeopathic treatment at a time, based on your specific symptoms. For information on homeopathy, see Chapter 4. For dosage information, see pages 56–57. Discontinue use if the symptoms disappear.

- Arnica (*Arnica montana*) 30c: Use when the gout-affected joint feels bruised. One dose every 15 minutes, for up to four doses.
- Colchicum (*Colchicum autumnale*) 6c: Use when the affected joint is excruciatingly painful and the person feels weak and nauseated. One dose every 15 minutes, for up to three hours.
- Ledum (*Ledum palustre*) 6c: Use when joints are swollen and feel cold; the pain eases with cold treatment and grows worse with movement. One dose every 15 minutes, for up to three hours.
- Urtica (*Urtica wrens*) 30c: Use when the affected

joints itch and burn. One dose every 15 minutes, for up to four doses.

An Ounce of Prevention

Lose weight, if necessary. Trimming down to your ideal body weight lowers uric acid levels in the blood, reducing your risk of a gout attack. Also, watch what you eat. Take special care to eliminate from your diet alcohol and foods containing purines.

Warning Signs

Gout usually strikes in the middle of the night, often after a night of overindulgence in food and drink. While it can take years for uric acid to build in the body before a gout outbreak, your body won't give you any warning of an impending attack.

For More Information:

Arthritis Foundation
1314 Spring Street, N.W.
Atlanta, GA 30309
(404) 872-7100
(800) 283-7800

National Arthritis and Musculoskeletal and Skin Diseases Information Clearinghouse
9000 Rockville Pike
P.O. Box AMS
Bethesda, MD 20892-2903
(301) 495-4484

American College of Rheumatology
60 Executive Park South, Suite 150
Atlanta, GA 30329
(404) 633-3777

Hair Loss

As the years go by, most of us tend to lose hair where we want it and grow hair where we don't. In what may seem like a cruel hoax, Mother Nature has arranged things so that the hormonal changes associated with aging cause a decrease in hair growth on the scalp and an increase in growth in the nostrils, ears, eyebrows, and other less favorable locations.

Heredity is the leading cause of hair loss, but most people—especially men—tend to lose their hair as they grow older. By age 60, most men have some degree of hair thinning or baldness. And about two-thirds of men have male-pattern baldness, a genetic condition that involves a sensitivity to androgens—male hormones that cause hair follicles to shut down. Pattern baldness can be passed down by either parent or grandparents.

In men, hair loss usually begins on either side of the forehead and at the crown of the head. In some cases it affects men as early as age 20, though it usually doesn't become apparent until the thirties. Women can also develop pattern baldness, though they generally lose hair more evenly, without a receding hairline or bald spots, and they usually hold on to their hair until after menopause.

In addition, hair loss—both temporary and permanent—can be caused or exacerbated by a number of medications, including drugs for hypertension, high cholesterol, arthritis, and ulcers. And of course, chemotherapy used in the treatment of cancer also causes dramatic hair loss. Other contributing factors include poor circulation, acute illness or trauma, surgery, skin disease, sudden weight loss, poor diet, iron or vitamin deficiency, diabetes, thyroid disease, hormonal disorders, and stress.

When it comes to hair loss, plenty of charlatans hawk specialized nostrums and elixirs that promise to grow a thick head of youthful hair—but most of the promises amount to little more than bald-faced lies. Still, there are natural remedies you can try to slow or perhaps even halt hair loss.

Conventional Care

When it comes to treating hair loss, medical doctors have several prescription drugs at their disposal, but only one—minoxidil (marketed under the name Rogaine)—has been approved by the Food and Drug Administration for treatment of baldness. (Minoxidil became available over-the-counter in 1996.) But the track record with minoxidil is less than impressive: Only one out of four men and one out of five women will grow any hair at all on the drug, and very few will experience dense growth. It is also expensive—about $30 a month—and it must be used twice a day, every day, for as long as you want to keep your new hair.

Another alternative is cosmetic surgery, including hair transplants, scalp lifts, and hair flaps, to change the appearance of the hairline. But these methods often cost thousands of dollars, and they do not always yield the desired results. And of course, there is a risk of infection, as is true with any surgery.

The Natural Approach

All of the natural remedies listed below can be used to supplement conventional medical treatment.

Herbal Medicine

Use one or more of the remedies listed below. For more information on herbal medicine, see Chapter 2. Commercial preparations are also available; follow package directions.

- Arnica *(Arnica montana):* This herb can be used to stimulate blood circulation to the scalp. Apply it as a cream or ointment to the scalp, or use a diluted tincture as a hair rinse. Do not use on broken skin. Tinctures and ointments are commercially available; follow package directions.
- Southernwood *(Artemisia abrotanum):* A hair rinse made from an infusion of this herb has long been used to stimulate hair growth. Commercially prepared tinctures are available use; follow package directions.

Diet and Nutrition Supplements

For information on nutrition supplements and good food sources of particular nutrients, see Chapter 3.

- Vitamin C: This vitamin helps improve blood circulation to the scalp. Take up to 3,000 milligrams a day, in divided doses.

Homeopathy

Use one homeopathic treatment at a time, based on your specific symptoms. For information on homeopathy, see Chapter 4. For dosage information, see pages 56–57. Discontinue use if the symptoms disappear.

- Baryta carb. *(Baryta carbonica)* 6c: Use if hair loss is in an older person with poor circulation. One dose twice a day, for up to four weeks.
- Lycopodium *(Lycopodium clavatum)* 6c: Use for premature hair loss or graying. Take one dose twice a day, for up to four weeks.
- Phosphorus *(Phosphorus)* 6c: Use when hair falls out in handfuls. One dose twice a day, for up to four weeks.
- Selenium *(Selenium)* 6c: Use when hair loss occurs both on the scalp and elsewhere on the body. One dose twice a day, for up to four weeks.

Acupressure

Use one or more of the acupressure points listed below. For information on acupressure, see Chapter 5. For diagrams showing the specific pressure points, see pages 88–91.

- Gallbladder 8: Just inside the hairline, two finger-widths above the top of the ears.
- Gallbladder 20: At the back of the head, in the depression between the base of the skull and the neck muscles.
- Governing Vessel 20: At the top of the head, straight up from the top of the ears.
- Kidney 3: On the inside of the ankle, in the depression next to the tip of the anklebone.

An Ounce of Prevention

Alas, if you're genetically destined to be bald, there are few steps you can take to halt the natural progression—but you may be able to slow it down. Hair loss caused by medication, excessive intake of vitamin A, or hair abuse—too much bleaching, teasing, straightening, curling, braiding, and perming—can be reversed by eliminating the cause of the temporary problem.

Warning Signs

Common hair loss is a gradual process that usually takes place over a number of years. But if your hair loss is sudden, spotty, or irregular, or if it is accompanied by a rash or scaly patches, contact your doctor. This type of hair loss can be a symptom of another health problem, such as ringworm or a dermatological disorder.

For More Information:

American Hair Loss Council
401 North Michigan Avenue, 22nd Floor
Chicago, IL 60611-4212
(800) 274-8717

Going Gray

A headful of gray hair is one of the most conspicuous signs of aging, but it is not always the most accurate. While most people start to show patches of gray hair between the ages of 30 and 40, some people begin graying before they turn 20—and others never do. In fact, one out of every three people has little or no gray at age 65 (even without the assistance of hair tints and coloring agents).

While we refer to hair as turning gray, it actually turns white. The gray color is an optical illusion caused by the mixture of the naturally colored hair with strands that have turned white. These white strands are caused by the loss of cells in the scalp that produce melanin, a pigment that gives color to the hair and skin. Though it varies from person to person, graying usually begins at the temples, then spreads to the crown and the back of the head. In men, the beard often turns gray first, and for most people, hair in the armpits and eyebrows changes last.

People with premature graying usually inherit the condition, though it can be triggered by severe emotional stress, malnutrition, or cardiovascular or autoimmune disease. While gray hair alone has no known health consequences, recent research suggests that people who gray early may also be prone to dangerously low bone mass. (The link between gray hair and bone mass remains unclear, though researchers suspect that the gray-hair gene may be located next to the genes involved in building bone mass.)

Most of us equate gray hair with old age, but fortunately there is a quick, easy, and inexpensive way to turn back the clock: Dye your hair.

Hearing Loss

As we grow older, the cumulative effect of a lifetime of noise takes its toll on our ears. That should come as no surprise when you consider that the human ear is a remarkably delicate organ. Sound waves enter the ear, causing minute vibrations on the eardrum. These vibrations stimulate the movement of tiny hairs in the inner ear; the hairs in turn convert these movements into nerve impulses, which are then transmitted to the brain by the auditory nerve. Then at last the brain receives the signal and registers sound. As we age, the tiny hairs deteriorate and don't conduct sound vibrations as well as they once did, causing hearing loss.

Age-related hearing loss (known as *presbycusis,* from the Greek meaning "old hearing") often begins in the twenties, but the changes are so subtle that they usually go unnoticed until age 60 or so, when loss of middle- and low-frequency hearing makes it difficult to discern speech.

Fully 60 percent of people over age 65 and 90 percent of those over age 75 have some hearing loss.

In addition to damage to the hairs, age can affect other structures in the ear. For example, the bones in the ear can become stiff and less responsive to vibration, and the eardrum itself may become thicker and less flexible. Some people also inherit a tendency for the bones in the ear to overgrow, causing other types of problems.

Hearing can also be compromised by other health problems, such as heart disease, high blood pressure, diabetes, and other circulatory disorders that can diminish the blood supply to the ears, causing damage. Acute ear infections can also damage the ear structure, leading to permanent hearing loss.

There are three types of hearing loss: conductive, sensorineural, and central deafness.

- Conductive hearing loss is caused by a blockage in the inner ear, usually earwax packed into the ear canal. Infection, fluid in the inner ear, and abnormal bone growth can also cause this type of hearing loss. Symptoms include voices sounding muffled while your own voice sounds loud; it may be accompanied by tinnitus, or ringing, hissing, buzzing, or clicking sounds in the ears.
- Sensorineural hearing loss is caused by problems with the acoustic nerve in the inner ear. In most cases people with this type of damage have trouble understanding speech but remain sensitive to loud sounds; they may also experience tinnitus. Sensorineural hearing loss can be the result of aging, exposure to loud noises, or a reaction to certain medications, such as aspirin, some antibiotics, and antihypertensive drugs. If a noise is exceptionally loud (such as an explosion), it can destroy the hairs outright. At somewhat lower levels (a rock concert or a car stereo at full blast, for example), the damage can be slow and steady.
- Central deafness is a rare condition caused by damage to the hearing centers of the brain. The person can

hear normally but cannot understand what is heard. This condition can be caused by stroke, prolonged high fever, or a blow to the head.

Conventional Care

Once a hearing problem is detected, treatment may involve the use of a hearing aid or other listening device, surgery to correct a physical problem, or training in lip reading to compensate for the lack of hearing.

Words of Wisdom

"Many people experience temporary hearing loss due to earwax buildup. Though many people don't realize it, chronic earwax buildup can be a symptom of food allergy. They clean out their ears, but the problem returns again and again. You have to look at the cause of the hearing problem."

Pam Taylor, N.D. B.A.
Moline, Illinois

The Natural Approach

All of the natural remedies listed below can be used to supplement conventional medical treatment.

Herbal Medicine

For more information on herbal medicine, see Chapter 2.

- Gingko *(Ginkgo biloba)*: The herb helps with hearing loss caused by decreased blood flow to the nerves in the ears. It is also useful in treating tinnitus. Commercial preparations are widely available; follow package directions.

Homeopathy

Use one homeopathic treatment at a time, based on your specific symptoms. For information on homeopathy, see Chapter 4. For dosage information, see pages 56–57. Discontinue use if the symptoms disappear.

- Chenopodium *(Chenopodium anthelminticum)* 6c: Use when hearing loss seems to be associated with aging and no other external factors. One dose four times a day, for up to one week.
- China *(China officinalis)* 6c: Use when hearing problems are associated with ringing, buzzing, humming, or roaring in the ears. One dose four times a day, for up to one week.
- Graphites *(Graphites)* 6c: Use when hearing improves when there is background noise. One dose four times a day, for up to one week.
- Phosphorus *(Phosphorus)* 6c: Use when it is difficult to separate voices from background noise. One dose four times a day, for up to one week.

Acupressure

Use one or more of the acupressure points listed below. For information on acupressure, see Chapter 5. For diagrams showing the specific pressure points, see pages 88–91.

- Bladder 23: On the lower back, two finger-widths on either side of the spine, approximately level with the waist. This point is particularly effective at reducing tinnitus.
- Gallbladder 2: Just behind the jawbone and in front of the lobe of the ear, in the depression formed when the mouth is open.
- Small Intestine 19: Just in front of the middle of the ear, in the depression formed when the mouth is slightly open.
- Triple Warmer 5: On the outside of the forearm, three

finger-widths above the wrist, in the hollow between the bones.

- Triple Warmer 21: In the depression in front of the notch at the top of the ear. The depression will deepen when the mouth is opened.

An Ounce of Prevention

The best way to protect your hearing is to avoid bombarding your ears with loud noises, which can cause permanent damage to the middle ear. The level of noise considered to be damaging is 85 to 90 decibels, lower than most people realize (normal speech is usually 65 to 70 decibels). If you listen to loud music, work around loud machinery, or use many everyday appliances such as vacuum cleaners and lawn mowers, you may be exposed to excessive noise. So-called "impulse noises," such as explosions from firearms or firecrackers, are particularly dangerous because they are so sudden. If you are going to be exposed to loud noises, wear protective earplugs, which are sold in drugstores and sporting goods stores.

You can also prevent hearing loss by taking care of ear infections promptly. Left untreated, an infection of the middle ear can cause permanent hearing loss. The problem can usually be cleared up with a ten-day course of antibiotics.

You can also avoid some hearing problems by getting your hearing checked regularly. Between the ages of 50 and 64, have a hearing exam at least once every five years. After age 65 have your primary care physician test your hearing as part of your regular annual physical exam.

A simple but crude test to measure high-frequency hearing loss is to rub your thumb and forefinger together near your ear. if you can't hear the rubbing sound, your hearing may be impaired.

Warning Signs

If you experience dizziness, pain, nausea, ringing in the ear, or sudden hearing loss in one or both ears, you should see a doctor. The problem could be a simple buildup of wax in the ear, or a more severe problem.

For More Information:

American Speech-Language-Hearing Association
10801 Rockville Pike
Rockville, MD 20852
(301) 897-5700; (301) 897-8682
(800) 638-8255

Better Hearing Institute
5021-B Backlick Road
Annandale, VA 22003
(800) EAR-WELL

International Hearing Society
20361 Middlebelt Road
Livonia, MI 48152
(810) 478-2610

National Information Center on Deafness
Gallaudet University
Health Department
800 Florida Avenue, N.E.
Washington, DC 20002

National Institute on Deafness and Other Communication Disorders Clearinghouse
1 Communication Avenue
Bethesda, MD 20892-3456
(800) 241-1044
(800) 241-1055 (TDD)

SHHH (Self Help for Hard of Hearing People, Inc.)
7910 Woodmont Avenue, Suite 1200
Bethesda, MD 20814
(301) 657-2248
(301) 657-2249 (TDD)

For free information on hearing problems or a free over-the-phone hearing test, call:
(800) 222-EARS
(800) 345-EARS (in Pennsylvania)

Do You Need a Hearing Aid?

Hearing aids help millions of people hear sounds and conversations they would otherwise miss out on, but they do not work for everyone.

Hearing aids, which can cost from about $400 for an off-the-shelf model to more than $2,000 for a state-of-the-art aid, do little more than amplify sound. They consist of a microphone to pick up the sound, an amplifier to make it louder, a receiver to transmit the sound to the ear, a battery for power, and a dial for volume control. All of this fits into a compact unit that can fit in the ear, behind the ear, or onto the frame of a pair of eyeglasses.

The problem with hearing aids is that as the sound is made louder, it becomes somewhat distorted. And because hearing aids amplify all the sound in the room, they work well in one-on-one conversation but can be confusing in a group setting, where an individual voice may be lost in the overall sound in the room.

It takes time to adjust to using a hearing aid. The best way to become accustomed to one is to wear it every day. Before buying a hearing aid, make sure you can return it within 30 days for a full refund if it does not improve your hearing sufficiently or if you are uncomfortable with it.

Be sure to deal with a reputable hearing specialist. There are a number of different types of hearing professionals, each with a different level of expertise:

- **Otologists or otolaryngologists** are medical doctors or doctors of osteopathy with extensive training in ear and hearing problems. They can diagnose and treat hearing disorders and perform surgery.

- **Audiologists** are licensed to conduct hearing tests and dispense hearing aids; they do not prescribe drugs or perform surgery. Audiologists should be certified by the American Speech-Language-Hearing Association; the initials CCC-A after their name indicate a Certificate of Clinical Competence in Audiology.
- **Hearing aid specialists** conduct hearing evaluations for the purpose of selling and fitting hearing aids; in most states they are not licensed, and they may or may not be adequately trained.

Now Hear This

Warning: When it comes to hearing loss, the danger zone begins at a lower volume than many people think. Hearing damage can occur at 80 to 85 decibels (dB); in fact the federal Occupational Safety and Health Administration (OSHA) requires employers to protect workers from extended noise levels of 85 dB and above.

How loud is loud? The following table can provide a general frame of reference:

Firearm	140 to 170 dB
Jet engine	140 dB
Rock concert	90 to 130 dB
Amplified car stereo	140 dB (full volume)
Portable stereo (Walkman)	115 dB (full volume)
Power mower	105 dB
Jackhammer	100 dB
Subway train	100 dB
Video arcade	100 dB

Freeway driving in a convertible	95 dB
Power saw	95 dB
Electric razor	85 dB
Crowded school bus	85 dB
School recess / assembly	85 dB
Garbage disposal	85 dB

Heart Attack and Cardiovascular Disease

Your heart and circulatory system feed every cell in your body with life-giving oxygen. This complex 12,400-mile network of arteries, veins, and blood vessels circulates blood from your heart to the farthest reaches of your body. In a healthy adult, the heart beats about 100,000 times a day, pumping the equivalent of more than 4,000 gallons of blood. That's an impressive accomplishment—one that underscores the importance of maintaining a well-tuned heart and circulatory system.

But all too often the system fails. Heart attacks, atherosclerosis, congestive heart failure, strokes, and other circulatory diseases claim about one million lives a year. In addition, a huge number of Americans—more than 63 million—live with some form of heart or blood vessel disease. Heart disease kills more people than any other ailment.

Although the risk of heart attack and cardiovascular disease increases with age, about a fifth of the deaths occur among people under age 65. Fortunately, many of these deaths can be prevented by lifestyle changes and by avoiding or minimizing the factors that raise the risk of cardiovascular disease.

Heart Attack

The heart is a muscle, and like any other muscle it needs oxygen to stay alive. When all or part of the heart muscle dies due to lack of oxygen, it is called a heart attack, or *myocardial infarction*. Each year more than 1.5 million Americans suffer heart attacks, and about one out of three of them dies.

Many heart attacks are caused by blood clots. When blood flows through an artery of the heart that has been narrowed by atherosclerosis, it slows down and tends to clot. When the clot becomes big enough, it cuts off the blood supply to the portion of the heart muscle below the clot, and that part of the heart muscle begins to die.

Heart attack can also occur when the heartbeat becomes irregular. In severe cases this condition, known as arrhythmia, can prevent sufficient blood from reaching the heart muscle.

Atherosclerosis

"Hardening of the arteries," or atherosclerosis, involves the gradual buildup of fatty deposits, or plaque in the arteries. The deposits narrow the arteries, reducing the blood supply to the heart and increasing the likelihood that a blood clot will clog up an arterial pathway and cause a heart attack.

Atherosclerosis is a three-step process. First, the arteries develop tiny tears due to the powerful contractions of the heart, especially in someone who has high blood pressure. Next, cholesterol in the blood sticks to the tears, slowly hardening into plaque, causing the arteries to become less flexible. Finally, these deposits narrow the arterial passages, reducing the blood supply to the heart muscle and other parts of the body.

The heart muscle is so efficient at extracting oxygen from the blood that many people develop severe coronary disease before any symptoms appear. In fact, the vessels can be 70 to 90 percent blocked before any symptoms occur—and often a heart attack is the first warning sign that something is wrong.

When it involves the coronary arteries, atherosclerosis causes heart attack. When it blocks blood flow to the brain, atherosclerosis causes stroke. And when it affects the arteries of the legs, it causes peripheral vascular disease.

Congestive Heart Failure

When the heart has been damaged and can no longer pump efficiently but has not failed outright, a person is suffering from congestive heart failure. When this occurs, the kidneys respond to the reduced blood circulation by retaining salt and water in the body, which adds additional stress to the heart and makes matters worse.

Congestive heart failure can affect either the right or left side of the heart. The left side pumps oxygen-rich blood from the lungs to the rest of the body. The right side of the heart pumps the oxygen-depleted blood back from the body to the lungs, where the oxygen is replenished. When the left side of the heart is damaged, the blood backs up in the lungs, causing wheezing and shortness of breath (even during rest), fatigue, sleep disturbances, and a dry, hacking, nonproductive cough when lying down. When the right side of the heart is damaged, the blood collects in the legs and liver, causing swollen feet and ankles, swollen neck veins, pain below the ribs, fatigue, and lethargy.

Stroke

A stroke is like a heart attack in the brain. Just as a part of the heart dies when deprived of oxygen during a heart attack, so a part of the brain dies when deprived of oxygen during a stroke. A *thrombotic stroke* occurs when an artery in the brain is blocked by a clot or atherosclerosis; an *embolic stroke* occurs when a small clot (known as an *embolus)* forms elsewhere in the body and moves to the brain, where it lodges in an artery and blocks the flow of blood. A *hemorrhagic stroke* occurs when an artery ruptures, usually due to high blood pressure. While hemorrhagic strokes are less common—only about 20 percent of all strokes—they are much more lethal, causing about 50 percent of all stroke-related deaths.

In the aftermath of a stroke, the person loses the bodily functions associated with the part of the brain that was destroyed. Symptoms of a stroke include slurred speech or loss of speech; sudden severe headache; double vision or blindness; sudden weakness or loss of sensation in the limbs; or loss of consciousness. These symptoms can occur over a period of a few minutes or hours, and they can occur on one side of the body or both.

Stroke is the nation's third leading cause of death and the leading cause of adult disability. Experts estimate that as many as 80 percent of all strokes can be prevented, either through changes in lifestyle or through the use of drugs to control high blood pressure and the tendency to form blood clots.

Conventional Care

Once cardiovascular disease is diagnosed, the goal of treatment is to halt—or even reverse—its progress. The strategy includes several tried and true lifestyle prescriptions: exercise (to strengthen the cardiovascular system), diet (to avoid artery-clogging foods), and weight control (to ease the workload on the heart). Steps should also be taken to lower blood cholesterol levels (see the box on pages 297–298).

Drugs may also be used to manage certain symptoms. Common medications used in the treatment of cardiovascular disease include nitroglycerine and other vasodilators (to open up the blood vessels); diuretics (to remove water from the body and reduce blood volume so that the heart doesn't have to work as hard); beta blockers (to inhibit the stress hormones adrenaline and noradrenaline, which cause the arteries to constrict); angiotensin inhibitors or ACE inhibitors (to block the reaction of certain enzymes that affect muscle contractions); and calcium-channel blockers (to inhibit the vessel-constricting calcium ions). In addition, old-fashioned aspirin is often prescribed to help thin the blood, reducing the risk of forming blood clots.

Still, despite the best efforts, coronary bypass surgery is sometimes required; each year nearly 200,000 Americans undergo the procedure. In a bypass operation segments of a healthy blood vessel (usually a vein from the leg) are grafted onto the heart's surface to bypass the clogged areas of the coronary arteries.

Another type of cardiovascular surgery is angioplasty, a procedure that uses a catheter and an inflatable balloon-like tip to flatten the fatty plaque deposits in the coronary arteries. Unfortunately, angioplasty does not work on all clogged coronary arteries; and good results can be temporary. Other less common treatments include heart transplants and the use of an experimental artificial heart.

Words of Wisdom

"We have compelling evidence about the ability of antioxidants—such as vitamin C and vitamin E—to reduce the risk of heart disease. Should people get antioxidants in their foods? Yes. Should they take supplements? Yes. There is no dichotomy between diet and supplements—you need both.

> Supplements are just that—they're supplements, not substitutes for a good diet."
>
> Jeffrey Blumberg, Ph.D.
> Professor of Nutrition
> Center on Aging,
> Tufts University
> Boston, Massachusetts

The Natural Approach

All of the natural remedies listed below can be used to supplement conventional medical treatment.

Herbal Medicine

Use one or more of the remedies listed below. For information on herbal medicine, see Chapter 2. Commercial preparations are also available; follow package directions.

- Dandelion *(Taraxacum officinale):* This diuretic herb helps lower blood pressure and relieves chronic liver congestion. Eat the fresh leaves in a salad or as a vegetable.
- Garlic *(Allium sativum):* This herb contains several sulfur compounds that block the biosynthesis of cholesterol. Garlic also helps expand the blood vessel walls, increasing blood flow and lowering blood pressure. Another chemical in garlic, ajoene, helps prevent blood clots. Use garlic liberally in cooking; eat up to 6 cloves of fresh garlic daily; or use commercially prepared odorless garlic capsules, available in health food stores.
- Ginkgo *(Ginkgo biloba):* This herb helps dilate the blood vessels and improves overall circulation. It is not generally available as a bulk herb, but it is available in commercial preparations.
- Hawthorn *(Crataegus oxyacantha):* This quintessential

"heart herb" enhances cardiac output, in addition to opening up the peripheral vessels to improve overall circulation. For an infusion, use 2 teaspoons of crushed leaves per cup of boiling water. Steep 20 minutes; strain, and drink up to two cups a day.

- Motherwort *(Leonurus cardiaca):* This herb calms heart palpitations and normalizes heart function in small doses. Commercial preparations are available at health food stores.
- Yarrow *(Achillea millefolium):* This herb acts as a diuretic by dilating peripheral blood vessels. It helps lower blood pressure and reduces pressure on the heart. Commercially prepared tinctures are available from health food stores.

Diet and Nutrition Supplements

What you eat may be a prime influence on the condition of your arteries and heart. Maintain a low-fat, low-sodium, high-fiber diet to prevent and recover from heart disease. Saturated fat encourages the body to produce cholesterol, which ends up as plaque on the arteries. To prevent heart disease, reduce fat intake to 20 to 30 percent of total caloric intake; to reverse heart disease, limit fat intake to 10 percent of calories. In addition, use one or more of the remedies listed below. For information on nutrition supplements and good food sources of particular nutrients, see Chapter 3.

- Calcium: Calcium is essential for blood clotting; it also plays a role in maintaining blood pressure. Take up to 1,500 milligrams a day.
- Fiber: A high-fiber diet helps lower cholesterol levels. The average American consumes only 11 grams of fiber a day, far short of the 25 grams experts recommend. If you don't care for high-fiber foods, take a psyllium-based supplement, following package directions. One study found that people who took one tablespoon of a soluble-fiber supplement twice a day for eight weeks had a 7 percent reduction in their low-

density lipoprotein (LDL) levels. (Fiber tablets won't provide the same cholesterol-lowering benefits, since they contain a synthetic insoluble fiber.)

- Folic acid: The body uses amino acids found in cow's milk and red meat to form homocysteine, an amino acid that helps create arterial lesions. Folic acid helps reduce homocysteine levels and lower the risk of heart disease. Take up to 400 milligrams a day.

- Magnesium: Magnesium is necessary to activate an enzyme that helps transport potassium to the cells. If the body lacks magnesium, and the potassium balance is disturbed, arrhythmias may result. Take up to 750 milligrams a day, or an amount equal to half your calcium supplement.

- Niacin: This vitamin plays an active role in more than fifteen metabolic reactions, most of which are important in the release of energy from carbohydrates. Niacin lowers the "bad" LDL cholesterol and triglycerides while raising the levels of high-density lipoproteins (HDLs), or "good" cholesterol. It also improves circulation by dilating the blood vessels. Check with your doctor before taking niacin. Take up to 50 milligrams a day, under your doctor's supervision. (At therapeutic doses niacin can cause liver damage, so your doctor should conduct periodic blood tests to monitor your liver function.)

- Potassium: Potassium, which is found in the intracellular fluids of the body, helps maintain cell integrity and water balance. It is also essential for muscle contraction and carbohydrate metabolism. Potassium is also an electrolyte and helps maintain the heart's electrical impulse and adequate heart rate. Take up to 5 grams a day.

- Soy: This protein contains two phytoestrogens—genistein and deidzen—that appear to help clear cholesterol from the blood. An analysis of 38 clinical trials found that people who ate an average of 47 grams of soy daily had a 13 percent drop in harmful LDL levels and a 9 percent drop in their total cholesterol. (Soy did not affect HDL levels.) Experts believe eating only 20 to 25 grams of soy daily—the equivalent of about 5 or 6 ounces of tofu—is enough to provide cholesterol-lowering benefits.

- Vitamin A: In addition to being powerful antioxidants, vitamin A and beta-carotene help to maintain elasticity in the tissues. Studies have shown that people who eat large amounts of beta-carotene have a significantly decreased mortality rate from cardiovascular disease, compared with those who don't eat much beta-carotene. The vitamin A in a multivitamin supplement should be sufficient.

- Vitamin C: This vitamin is essential for cholesterol metabolism. It is responsible for the excretion of excess cholesterol from the body, and it helps the body balance "good" and "bad" lipids, one of the biggest factors in heart disease. Take up to 3,000 milligrams a day, in divided doses.

- Vitamin E: This antioxidant helps prevent free radical damage, in addition to helping the body maintain cardiac and smooth muscle. It also keeps one particular form of LDL cholesterol from oxidizing and forming plaque deposits on the arteries. Take 400 to 800 IU a day.

Homeopathy

Use one homeopathic treatment at a time, based on your specific symptoms. For information on homeopathy, see Chapter 5. For dosage information, see pages 56–57. Discontinue use if the symptoms disappear.

- Aconite. *(Aconitum napellus)* 30c: Use when the person is frightened and afraid of dying in response to stroke or heart problem. One dose every 15 minutes, for up to ten doses while seeking medical help.

- Arnica *(Arnica montana)* 6c: Use immediately after stroke. One dose four times daily, for up to two weeks.

- Arsenicum iod. *(Arsenicum iodatum)* 6c: Use when

someone has advanced heart disease, arteriosclerosis, or fluid around the lungs. One dose four times daily, for up to three days.

- Baryta carb. *(Baryta carbonica)* 6c: Use when an elderly person suffers from high blood pressure and heart palpitations. One dose twice daily, for up to one month.
- Digitalis *(Digitalis purpurea)* 6c: Use when heart palpitations are brought on with the slightest exertion. One dose four times daily, for up to three days.
- Lachesis *(Trigonocephalus lachesis)* 6c: Use when the person has slow speech following a stroke. One dose four times daily, for up to three weeks.
- Nux *(Strychnos nux vomica)* 6c: Use at first sign of stroke. One dose every 15 minutes, for up to ten doses, while seeking medical help.
- Rhus tox. *(Rhus toxicodendron)* 6c: Use when the left arm feels numb and weak following a heart attack. One dose every 3 hours, for up to one week after the heart attack.

Acupressure

Use one or more of the acupressure points listed below. For information on acupressure, see Chapter 5. For diagrams showing the specific pressure points, see pages 88–91.

- Bladder 15: Two finger-widths out on either side of the spine, level with the fifth thoracic vertebra (approximately halfway between the shoulder blades). This point relieves heart palpitations and improves overall heart function.
- Conception Vessel 17: In the middle of the chest, in line with the nipples. This point helps relieve heart palpitations; it also improves heart and lung function.
- Heart 3: On the inside of the elbow, at the inside edge of the crease, when the elbow is flexed. This point relieves cardiac pain and constriction in the chest.
- Heart 7: With your palm facing upward, this point is

located on the outside edge of the wrist crease closest to the palm, in the hollow level with the little finger. This point improves circulation and strengthens the heart.

- Pericardium 4: On the inside of the forearm, halfway between the wrist and the elbow, in line with the middle finger, in the depression between the tendons. This point relieves cardiac pain and heart palpitations.
- Pericardium 6: This point is located three finger-widths above the wrist crease closest to the palm, between the tendons on the inside of the arm. This point relieves chest pain associated with angina, stimulates the heart function, and promotes good circulation, especially in the arms and chest.
- Stomach 36: Four finger-widths below the kneecap, on the outside edge of the leg bone (tibia). This point improves overall circulation.

An Ounce of Prevention

The major risk factors for heart disease and circulatory problems include smoking, high blood pressure, obesity, high blood cholesterol levels, and a family history of the disease. There are steps you can take to reduce many of these risks:

- Stop smoking. Smoking constricts the arteries, raises blood pressure, increases arterial tearing, speeds atherosclerosis, and reduces the oxygen levels in the blood. Smokers have two to four times the risk of heart attack as nonsmokers, and their heart attacks are more likely to be fatal. But there is hope: A decade after quitting, a former pack-a-day smoker has almost the same heart attack risk as if he or she had never smoked.
- Exercise to keep your arteries strong and flexible. Aerobic exercise helps prevent cardiovascular disease by lowering LDL cholesterol levels and raising HDL

cholesterol levels, reducing blood pressure, keeping weight down, burning fat, lowering blood-sugar levels, and boosting relaxation. People who exercise regularly are about half as likely as sedentary people to have a heart attack. Furthermore, people who exercised as part of their rehabilitation after a heart attack had a 25 percent reduction in second attacks. (For information on exercise, see Chapter 6.)

- Maintain healthy body weight. Excess body fat increases blood pressure and adds stress to the heart and circulatory system. People who maintain their ideal body weight are 35 to 55 percent less likely to have a heart attack than those who are obese (20 percent or more above their ideal weight).

- Become more aware of your anger, anxiety, and fear. These negative emotions trigger the release of adrenaline and increase blood pressure. These hormones also encourage the cells to release fat and cholesterol into the bloodstream. Defuse these emotions by practicing stress-management techniques (see Chapter 9).

- Review all prescription and over-the-counter drugs with your doctor. Some medications make your body retain more fluid, further straining your heart. Ask your doctor to assess the medications you're taking for possible adverse effects.

- Lower your blood cholesterol, if necessary. Elevated levels of blood cholesterol increase the risk of atherosclerosis. (See box on pages 297–298 for information on cholesterol.)

- Keep your blood pressure out of the danger zone. High blood pressure—a systolic reading above 140 millimeters of mercury (mm HG) and a diastolic reading above 90 mm Hg—is a major risk factor for heart attack. In general, for every one-point reduction in diastolic pressure, your heart attack rate falls by 2 to 3 percent. (For information on high blood pressure, or hypertension, see page 305.)

- Know your history. While there's nothing you can do to control your hereditary predisposition to cardiovascular disease, knowing your medical history can help you manage your risk factors. A family history of early heart attacks, high blood pressure, or stroke greatly increases your risk of developing cardiovascular disease. Anyone whose parents or other close relatives have suffered a heart attack or stroke before age 55 should make a special effort to minimize their other risk factors.

Warning Signs

Some people learn they have heart disease when they experience the chest-crushing pain of angina (see page 154 for more information). But many others don't receive any warning—until they have their first heart attack.

Heart attack victims often delay seeking medical help, frequently with fatal results. Most heart attack deaths occur in the first two hours, yet studies have found that many people wait four to six hours to get to an emergency room. Never ignore the warning signs of heart attack, including:

- Chest pain: an uncomfortable pressure, fullness, squeezing, or crushing feeling in the center of the chest that lasts two minutes or longer
- Severe pain that radiates to the shoulders, neck, arms, jaw, or top of the stomach
- Shortness of breath
- Paleness
- Sweating
- Rapid or irregular pulse
- Dizziness, fainting, or loss of consciousness

Not all of these warning signs occur in every heart attack. And some people, especially older people and diabetics, may not experience symptoms during a heart attack. (These so-called "silent heart attacks" can be detected only by an electrocardiogram.) If you suspect you may be experiencing a heart attack, get emergency medical help immediately. Doctors can prescribe a number of drugs that dissolve clots and reduce the oxygen demands of the heart, but these medications are most effective if given within one hour of the onset of a heart attack.

For More Information:

American Heart Association
7272 Greenville Avenue
Dallas, TX 75231
(214) 373-6300

Citizens for Public Action on Blood Pressure and Cholesterol
P.O. Box 30374
Bethesda, MD 20824
(301) 770-1711

International Atherosclerosis Society
6550 Fannin, No. 1423
Houston, TX 77030
(713) 790-4226

Mended Hearts
7272 Greenville Avenue
Dallas, TX 75231-4966
(214) 706-1442

National Heart Lung and Blood Institute
Information Center
National Institutes of Health
(301) 251-1222

National Heart Savers Association
9140 West Dodge Road
Omaha, NE 68114
(402) 398-1993

National Hypertension Association
324 East 30th Street
New York, NY 10016
(212) 889-3557

Cholesterol: The Numbers Game

The evidence is undeniable: Study after study has shown that the higher your levels of blood cholesterol, the greater your chances of dying from heart disease. Fortunately, the converse is also true: For every 1 percent you lower your total cholesterol level, you reduce your heart disease risk by 2 to 3 percent.

Your job is to find out your cholesterol levels—and then to figure out exactly what they mean. Generally speaking, the lower your total cholesterol levels, the better. A level below 200 milligrams/deciliter would be ideal. However, there's more to the story.

Before the cholesterol can enter the bloodstream, it must attach itself to a lipoprotein. (Cholesterol is a fatlike substance, and blood is essentially water; the lipoprotein is necessary to transport the cholesterol through the blood since fat and water don't mix.) There are two types of lipoproteins: low-density lipoproteins (LDLs) and high-density lipoproteins (HDLs). LDLs contribute to the formation of plaque deposits in the arteries, and HDLs help remove plaque deposits from the arteries.

Cardiovascular problems occur when the blood has too little HDL or too much LDL. As the table shows, you want to have low levels of LDL cholesterol and high levels of HDL cholesterol to minimize your risk of cardiovascular disease.

You can raise your HDLs by exercising and eating a diet rich in fruits and vegetables. For postmenopausal women, estrogen replacement therapy also helps (see pages 347–349 for information on hormone therapy).

To lower your LDL level, you must watch what you eat. The American Heart Association recommends limiting cholesterol intake to about 300 milligrams per day—the amount in one egg yolk. In addition, you should eat less fat in general, and less saturated fat in particular. Start by restricting your fat intake to no more than 30 percent of the calories from fat and only 10 percent from saturated fat. (That's 65 grams of fat and 22 grams of saturated fat for the average 2,000-calorie diet.) If your LDL levels don't fall within two or three months, cut the fat back to 20 percent of calories from fat and 7 percent from saturated fat. (Saturated fat is essentially animal fat, so it is especially high in cholesterol.)

You can also help to lower your LDL levels by eating more soluble fiber. For example, studies have found that adding a daily bowl of oat cereal can lower LDL cholesterol levels by 5 to 10 percent.

Though cholesterol has a bad reputation for clogging the arteries, don't think of it as the enemy. Cholesterol is actually essential for a number of vital bodily processes, including nerve function, reproduction, and the formation of cell membranes. While cholesterol is found in some of the foods we eat, most of it is manufactured by the liver. In fact, each day our bodies churn out about 1,000 milligrams of the waxy white stuff, compared to the average dietary intake of about 325 milligrams for men or 220 milligrams for women.

Cholesterol presents problems only when the supply exceeds the body's demand for it. Unneeded cholesterol circulates in the bloodstream, where it can stick to the walls of the arteries and form the fatty deposits known as plaque. These cholesterol deposits build up over time and eventually restrict the blood flow, causing cardiovascular disease. High cholesterol has also been implicated in causing gallstones, colon polyps, impotence, and high blood pressure. To avoid these problems, know your cholesterol levels and work to adjust them, if necessary.

WHAT DO YOUR NUMBERS MEAN?

	Desirable	Borderline	Undesirable
Total cholesterol			
	below 200	200–239	240 or higher
LDL cholesterol			
	below 130	130–159	160 or higher
HDL cholesterol	above 45	35–45	below 35
Ratio (total cholesterol/HDLs)	below 4.5	4.5–5.5	above 5.5

Hemorrhoids

Most people don't like to talk about them, but four out of five Americans experience hemorrhoids at some point in their lives. Hemorrhoids, those inflamed and widened veins that look like purple skin growths around the anus, can be painful, itchy—and embarrassing. While they affect people of all ages, about half of people over 50 experience hemorrhoids at any given time.

Hemorrhoids (also known as piles) can appear either outside or inside the anus. They can be caused by constipation, obesity, pregnancy, improper diet, lack of exercise, heavy lifting, prolonged periods of sitting, or liver damage. The condition tends to run in families, either because people inherit delicate veins or because they acquire similar lifestyles and personal habits that can exacerbate the problem. Either way, many cases of hemorrhoids can be prevented by carefully monitoring bowel function.

Conventional Care

Most doctors attempt to relieve discomfort of hemorrhoids by prescribing a high-fiber diet, increased fluid intake, and either suppositories, pads, or creams containing corticosteroid drugs to reduce the swelling and pain. In more severe cases, the hemorrhoidal tissue may need to be removed using liquid nitrogen, laser surgery, or traditional surgery.

Your doctor may recommend that you switch from toilet paper to premoistened tissues or baby wipes and that you take several sitz baths daily to provide both cleansing and relief. (For a sitz bath, sit in a warm bath of 4 to 6 inches of water for 5 to 15 minutes.) You may also be told to wear loose cotton underwear and clothing to allow air to circulate to the area.

Words of Wisdom

"Hemorrhoids are directly related to the fact that people don't observe the rule of one meal in, one meal out. To find out if your colon is working efficiently, you can test your colon transit time by eating a half cup of corn or a half cup of lightly steamed beets in the evening along with your regular meal. You should be able to see the corn and/or the color of the beets in the stools 12 to 18 hours later, preferably 12 hours. If it's longer, there's too much time for toxins to accumulate in the body; if it's more rapid, then there may be a problem with nutrient assimilation. When you correct the bowel problem, the hemorrhoids will disappear."

Jeanne Silk, R.N., M.A.
Co-owner, Body Balance Center
Lake Forest, California

The Natural Approach

All of the natural remedies listed below can be used to supplement conventional medical treatment.

Herbal Medicine

Use one or more of the remedies listed below. For information on herbal medicine, see Chapter 2. Commercial preparations are available; follow package directions.

- Blackberry *(Rubus fruticosus):* The astringent nature of blackberry has led to its use as a hemorrhoid treatment. For an infusion, use 2 to 3 teaspoons of dried leaves per cup of boiling water. Steep 10 to 20 minutes; drink up to three cups a day. You can also soak a clean cloth in a strong infusion and apply externally for 10 to 15 minutes two or three times a day.
- Pilewort *(Ranunculus ficaria):* Used topically, this astringent herb stops bleeding and heals blood vessels. Commercially prepared ointments are available from health food stores.
- Stoneroot *(Collinsonia canadensis):* This herb works exceptionally well on hemorrhoids, strengthening the veins and acting as an astringent. Powders and tinctures are commercially available from health food stores.
- Witch hazel *(Hamamelis virginiana):* Used topically, this herb will shrink blood vessels and stop minor bleeding. A witch hazel tincture or concentrated herbal drops are preferable to witch hazel liniments containing methyl or wood alcohol; witch hazel tinctures, herbal drops, and liniments can be found in conventional pharmacies and health food stores. Follow package directions. For extra relief, chill the preparation in the refrigerator before using.

Diet and Nutrition Supplements

Use one or more of the remedies listed below. For information on nutrition supplements and good food sources of particular nutrients, see Chapter 3.

- High-fiber diet. Hemorrhoids are rare in cultures where people eat a high-fiber diet. Eat plenty of whole grains and fresh fruits and vegetables.

- Water. To avoid constipation and keep stools soft, drink at least eight 8-ounce glasses—one gallon—of water a day. Keep in mind that caffeinated and alcoholic beverages do not count toward your fluid consumption goal. In fact, for every glass of caffeinated and alcoholic beverages you drink, you'll need to drink two glasses of water, because these drinks actually draw moisture away from the body.
- Zinc. To help reduce inflammation and promote tissue healing, take 50 milligrams of zinc a day.

Homeopathy

Use one homeopathic treatment at a time, based on your specific symptoms. For information on homeopathy, see Chapter 4. For dosage information, see pages 56–57. Discontinue use if the symptoms disappear.

- Aesculus *(Aesculus hippocastanum)* 6c: Use when hemorrhoids accompany constipation, and the stools are lumpy. One dose four times a day, for up to five days.
- Capsicum *(Capsicum annum)* 6c: Use when hemorrhoids protrude from the anus and burn. One dose four times a day, for up to five days.
- Hamamelis *(Hamamelis virginiana):* Use when hemorrhoids bleed or feel strained. One dose four times a day, for up to five days.
- Nitric ac. *(Nitricum acidum)* 6c: Use when anal fissures accompany hemorrhoids, and there is pain before, during, and after bowel movement. One dose four times a day, for up to five days.

Acupressure

Use one or more of the acupressure points listed below. For information on acupressure, see Chapter 5. For diagrams showing the specific pressure points, see pages 88–91.

- Large Intestine 4: On the outside of the hand, in the webbing between the thumb and index finger. The point is located at the highest spot of muscle when the thumb and index finger are brought together.
- Large Intestine 11: On the arm, at the outer edge of the elbow crease.
- Stomach 36: Four finger-widths below the kneecap and one finger-width outside the shinbone. (If you're in the right spot, you'll be able to feel your muscle flex as you move your foot up and down.)

An Ounce of Prevention

While some unfortunate people tend to be more susceptible to hemorrhoids than others, you can avoid many episodes by not straining or pushing during bowel movements. You can also prevent hemorrhoids in many cases by following the same regimen used to treat them—by drinking at least eight 8-ounce glasses of water a day and eating a high-fiber diet rich in fresh fruits and vegetables.

Warning Signs

If you develop hemorrhoids, you'll know it. Symptoms include rectal pain and tenderness, itching, and sometimes bleeding. In many cases the first—and most startling—sign of hemorrhoids is bright red blood in the stool, caused by pressure during the bowel movement. The bleeding is usually minor. But dark, tarry blood could indicate a more severe internal bleeding problem and should be brought to a medical doctor's attention immediately.

Hypertension

Listen up: If you have hypertension, your body is telling you something. Hypertension—or high blood pressure—is more than a medical annoyance; it is the most accurate predictor of future cardiovascular disease in people over age 65.

At the most basic level hypertension refers to the pressure of the blood against the blood vessels as the heart pumps it through the arteries. A blood pressure reading consists of two numbers: the systolic pressure (the higher number, reflecting the pressure when the heart contracts) and the diastolic pressure (the lower number, reflecting the pressure as the heart rests between beats). A normal blood pressure reading is 120/80, though the numbers fluctuate somewhat throughout the day. If your blood pressure is 140/90 or higher, you have hypertension and need to work on lowering it.

Hypertension cannot be cured, but it can—and must—

be controlled. Untreated, high blood pressure can lead to stroke, heart disease and heart attack, loss of vision, and kidney failure because the heart must work harder than normal to pump blood. In fact, people with hypertension face a risk of heart attack three times greater and a risk of stroke seven times greater than that of people with normal blood pressure.

High blood pressure is very common. Approximately one out of every ten Americans suffers from hypertension, including more than half of all older adults. Those at increased risk include African Americans, people who smoke, those who are overweight, and those who have a family history of hypertension. High blood pressure can also be caused by arteriosclerosis (hardening of the arteries), atherosclerosis (the formation of cholesterol plaque in the arteries), congestive heart failure, kidney disease, diabetes, pregnancy, and hormonal disorders.

Fortunately, in most cases high blood pressure can be lowered by diet and lifestyle changes. Hypertension should not be considered an inevitable consequence of aging; it can be controlled.

How High Is High?

Stage 1 hypertension:	Systolic pressure of 140–159
	Diastolic pressure of 90 to 99
Stage 2 hypertension:	Systolic pressure of 160 to 179
	Diastolic pressure of 100 to 109
Stage 3 hypertension:	Systolic pressure of 180 to 209
	Diastolic pressure of 110 to 119
Stage 4 hypertension:	Systolic pressure of 210 or more
	Diastolic pressure of 120 or more

Conventional Care

To assess the potential damage caused by hypertension, a physician may order a number of tests, including an EKG (to see if there has been any damage to the heart), a chest X ray (to find out if the heart has been enlarged), a urinalysis (to determine if protein or red blood cells are present in the urine, indicating kidney damage), and a blood test (to assess kidney function). In most cases these tests provide enough information to outline a treatment program involving diet and lifestyle changes and often drug therapy. Common antihypertensive drugs include diuretics, beta-blockers, alpha-blockers, angiotensin-converting enzyme (ACE) inhibitors, calcium-channel blockers, and vasodilators. African Americans tend to respond well to diuretics and calcium-channel blockers, but not as well to beta-blockers and other antihypertensive drugs.

In addition, you may be asked to buy a blood pressure monitor and learn to take your own blood pressure so that you can chart your levels on a regular basis. This will help you evaluate the effectiveness of the drug therapy, as well as allow you to keep an eye on your overall levels.

Words of Wisdom

"Hypertension is a silent disease: If you don't control it, hypertension will destroy your kidneys, damage your blood vessels, and strain your heart— and a cascade of dangerous consequences will follow. It can be a difficult problem to manage because there are probably thirty different causes of hypertension, and what is an important factor in one individual may not be important in another. There are also a number of cases where there is no obvious cause that can be identified. You may have to try different treatments to find one that works, but it is absolutely essential that you identify the problem and take some steps to treat it."

Oliver Alabaster, M.D.
Director, Institute for Disease Prevention
George Washington University

The Natural Approach

All of the natural remedies listed below can be used to supplement conventional medical treatment.

Herbal Medicine

Use one or more of the remedies listed below. For information on herbal medicine, see Chapter 2. Commercial preparations are also available; follow package directions.

- Barberry *(Berberis vulgaris):* Barberry lowers blood pressure by enlarging the blood vessels. For a decoction, use 1/2 teaspoon of powdered root bark boiled in a cup of water for 15 minutes. Drink one cup a day. Commercial preparations are also available; follow package directions.
- Celery *(Apium graveolens):* Eating celery (as well as consuming celery oil and celery seeds) helps to lower blood pressure by relaxing the smooth muscles in the blood vessels. Chomping on as few as four stalks of celery a day provides enough of the active ingredient,

a compound known as 3-butylphthalide, to reduce blood pressure.

- Garlic *(Allium sativum):* Garlic is a powerful blood-pressure-lowering agent—it has been shown to lower the systolic pressure by an impressive 20 to 30 mm Hg and the diastolic by 10 to 20 mm Hg. Consume 3 to 10 cloves of fresh garlic a day, or use commercial garlic preparations, following package directions.
- Hawthorn *(Crataegus oxyacantha):* Widely used in Europe, hawthorn lowers blood pressure, improves coronary circulation, prevents cholesterol deposits from forming on artery walls, and helps strengthen the heart muscle. Commercially prepared infusions and tinctures are available; follow package directions.
- Yarrow *(Achillea millefolium):* This herb improves blood flow and lowers blood pressure by relaxing the peripheral blood vessels. Commercially prepared tinctures are available; follow package directions.

Diet and Nutrition Supplements

Use one or more of the remedies listed below. Some vitamins can be used topically, as noted. For information on nutrition supplements and good food sources of particular nutrients, see Chapter 3.

- Calcium and magnesium: Low levels of calcium and magnesium can contribute to hypertension. Fortunately, supplements and increased dietary intake help reverse the condition. Take 1,500 milligrams of calcium and 750 milligrams of magnesium a day.
- Coenzyme Q-10: People with hypertension tend to be deficient in coenzyme Q-10 (also called CoQ-10), an essential component in the metabolic process of energy production. It appears that the enzyme helps regulate blood pressure and strengthens the walls of the blood vessels. Coenzyme Q-10 is available commercially; follow package directions.
- High-fiber diet: A diet high in fiber has been shown to prevent and treat hypertension and other forms of

cardiovascular disease. Change your overall diet as necessary to increase your intake of fiber, especially soluble gel-forming fibers such as oat bran, apple pectin, and psyllium seeds.

- Potassium: Low levels of potassium, especially when combined with high levels of sodium, increase fluid retention and inhibit the body's blood-pressure-regulating system. A diet high in potassium and low in sodium lowers blood pressure, partially by reducing the blood-vessel-constricting property of adrenaline. Unfortunately, limiting sodium alone won't necessarily control hypertension; you need to combine low sodium with high potassium in your diet.

- Vitamin C: Several studies have shown that the lower the levels of vitamin C, the higher a person's blood pressure. One study found that taking as little as 250 milligrams of vitamin C a day slashed the risk of high blood pressure by almost half. Take 1 to 1 1/2 grams of vitamin C daily.

Foods to Avoid

The sodium in salt (sodium chloride) makes the body retain fluids, which in turn raises blood pressure and forces your heart to work harder. About 70 percent of our sodium intake comes from processed foods. Read all food labels carefully, keeping an eye out for foods containing "soda," "sodium," or the symbol "Na" on the label. In addition, avoid high-sodium foods such as smoked or aged cheeses and meats, chocolate, animal fats, tomato juice, canned soups and vegetables, gravy, bouillon, and processed foods. As many as half of all hypertensives are particularly salt sensitive and will benefit from reducing their sodium intake.

Homeopathy

For information on homeopathy, see Chapter 4. For dosage information, see pages 56–57. Discontinue use if the symptoms disappear.

- Baryta carb. *(Baryta carbonica)* 6c: Use if the person suffers from high blood pressure and heart palpitations. One dose twice a day, for up to four weeks.

Acupressure

Use one or more of the acupressure points listed below. For information on acupressure, see Chapter 5. For diagrams showing the specific pressure points, see pages 88–91.

- Governing Vessel 16: In the center of the back of the head, in the large hollow under the base of the skull.
- Kidney 1: A third of the way down the sole of the foot, in the depression just below the ball of the foot.
- Liver 3: On the top of the foot, in the valley between the big toe and the second toe.

An Ounce of Prevention

Not every case of hypertension can be controlled or prevented by lifestyle changes, but many can be. Keep the following tips in mind:

- Know your blood pressure. If your numbers are borderline or elevated (140/90 or higher), then contact your physician and recheck your levels at least once a month.
- Don't smoke, and avoid being around people who do. Nicotine constricts arteries and elevates blood pressure. A person with uncontrolled hypertension who smokes is five times more likely to have a heart attack and sixteen times more likely to have a stroke than a nonsmoker.
- Exercise regularly. Aerobic exercise three times a week for 20 to 30 minutes can improve cardiovascular health and lower blood pressure.
- Lose weight, if necessary. People who are overweight tend to experience more hypertension. (For informa-

tion on weight loss, see Chapter 8.) About half of all people with hypertension are overweight. An analysis of five studies involving weight loss and hypertension found that, on average, losing 20 pounds resulted in a decline of 6.3 mm Hg in systolic and 3.1 mm Hg in diastolic pressure.

- Monitor your use of over-the-counter medicines. Avoid using over-the-counter antihistamines, decongestants, cold remedies, and appetite suppressants, unless recommended by your doctor. These drugs can raise blood pressure.
- Try to manage your daily stress. Stress can temporarily elevate blood pressure. Relaxation techniques such as biofeedback, meditation, yoga, progressive muscle relaxation, and hypnosis have been show to help lower blood pressure (for information on stress reduction, see Chapter 9). Some researchers suspect that prolonged exposure to stress can cause a permanent rise in blood pressure.
- Avoid coffee and caffeinated beverages, which can elevate blood pressure.
- Restrict alcohol consumption. While some researchers tout the cardiovascular benefits of modest drinking, consuming more than 30 milliliters of alcohol a day—an amount equal to 1 ounce of 100-proof whiskey, 8 ounces of wine, or two 12-ounce beers—can raise blood pressure.

Warning Signs

Hypertension is often called "the silent killer" because it strikes without warning. About 20 percent of Americans with high blood pressure don't know they have the condition, and only one-third have it under control. Advanced hypertension can sometimes cause headache (especially in the morning), fatigue, dizziness, rapid pulse, shortness of breath, sweating, nosebleeds, and visual problems. The only way to be sure your blood pressure is under control is to visit your doctor regularly and have your blood pressure checked. If you suffer from hypertension, you need to be under the care of a physician who can monitor this potentially life-threatening condition.

For More Information:

National Heart, Lung, and Blood Institute
Information Center
National Institutes of Health
(301) 251-1222

National Hypertension Association
324 East 30th Street
New York, NY 10016
(212) 889-3557

American Society of Hypertension
515 Madison Avenue, Suite 1212
New York, NY 10022
(212) 644-0650

Citizens for Public Action on Blood Pressure and Cholesterol
P.O. Box 30374
Bethesda, MD 20824
(301) 770-1711

Hysterectomy

Hysterectomy should not be taken lightly, even if a woman is well past her childbearing years. The procedure, which involves the surgical removal of the uterus, affects overall health and sexuality in a number of ways. Hysterectomy alters the delicate hormonal balance in the body, even if the ovaries are left intact. Though many women assume the uterus is of little importance following menopause, in truth it continues to release hormones and to interact with other hormones in the body well after the end of menstruation. These changes in hormone levels can increase the risk of osteoporosis and heart disease; they also contribute to vaginal dryness, mood changes, and hot flashes (see the section on menopause, page 340).

Despite the disadvantages associated with the procedure, one out of every three American women has a hysterectomy by the age of 60. While hysterectomy is unquestionably necessary in many cases—such as bleeding combined with anemia, fibroid tumors that block bowel or urinary function, severe endometriosis, reproductive cancers, or advanced pelvic inflammatory disease, among others—many of the operations are not clearly necessary. In fact, only an estimated 8 to 12 percent of hysterectomies are performed to treat cancer and other life-threatening illnesses.

Depending on your specific medical needs, there are several different types of hysterectomy: partial hysterectomy (only the uterus is removed), total hysterectomy (the uterus and cervix are removed); and pan hysterectomy (the uterus, ovaries, and fallopian tubes are removed). The most dramatic consequences occur when the ovaries are removed, eliminating the body's source of estrogen and causing instant menopause. Always seek a second opinion, and when surgery is necessary, consider using a number of natural remedies that can be helpful during recovery.

Conventional Care

A hysterectomy is major surgery, requiring up to two months for recovery, depending on your age and overall health. After the operation, many women go through a difficult period of adjustment due to hormonal and psychological changes associated with a perceived "loss of femininity" caused by the removal of this important reproductive organ.

Words of Wisdom

"Having a hysterectomy is very disruptive to a woman's body. After the operation, her estrogen levels drop, leaving her susceptible to a number of problems, including osteoporosis. To avoid the brittle bones of osteoporosis, a woman who has had a hysterectomy should be sure to take calcium supplements—something many women neglect to do."

JoAnne Williams, N.D.
Miami, Florida

The Natural Approach

The natural remedies listed below cannot prevent a hysterectomy if one is medically 'necessary. But they can help heal the body after the procedure and during the difficult postsurgical period of hormonal adjustment. All of the natural remedies listed below can be used to supplement conventional medical treatment. In addition, see the menopause section on page 340 for information on how to manage some of the hormonal changes associated with hysterectomy.

Herbal Medicine

Use one or more of the remedies listed below. For information on herbal medicine, see Chapter 2. Commercial preparation are also available; follow package directions.

- Basil *(Ocimum basilicum):* This herb can elevate mood and reverse the depression associated with hormonal changes before—and after—a hysterectomy. Eat two or three fresh basil leaves with salads, or take a commercially prepared tincture, following package directions.
- Wood betony *(Stachys officinalis):* To ease anxiety and calm the body as it undergoes the difficult hormonal changes associated with hysterectomy, use a commercially prepared infusion or tincture of wood betony. Follow package directions.

Diet and Nutrition Supplements

Use one or more of the remedies listed below. For information on nutrition supplements and good food sources of particular nutrients, see Chapter 3.

- Calcium and magnesium: Estrogen helps the body absorb calcium, which is necessary for strong bones and to ward off osteoporosis. When estrogen levels drop after hysterectomy, absorption of these minerals is impaired, so supplements may be necessary. Take 1,500 milligrams of calcium and 750 milligrams of magnesium a day.

- Vitamin E: This vitamin helps with estrogen production and eases hot flashes associated with menopause or the hormonal changes after hysterectomy. Take 400 IU daily.

Homeopathy

Use one homeopathic treatment at a time, based on your specific symptoms. For information on homeopathy, see Chapter 4. For dosage information, see pages 56–57. Discontinue use if the symptoms disappear.

- Arnica *(Arnica montana)* 30c: Use immediately after a hysterectomy to minimize pain and promote healing. One dose per hour for the first three hours, then twice a day for up to five days.
- Staphisagria *(Delphinium staphisagria)* 6c: Use if the healing after a hysterectomy is slow, or if there are any surgical complications. One dose four times a day, for up to five days.

An Ounce of Prevention

Doctors often debate the pros and cons of elective hysterectomy. Some advocates argue that too many physicians opt for surgery when less invasive methods can be used; others counter that hysterectomy can prevent many health problems. While some hysterectomies are undoubtedly necessary, surgery may not be the best solution for all women with abnormal uterine bleeding, mild fibroids, endometriosis, or uterine prolapse. These problems cannot be prevented, but there may be other nonsurgical treatments that should be tried before surgery is considered.

Warning Signs

A hysterectomy is a planned surgical procedure. Nearly 600,000 American women undergo it each year. Be sure to discuss the pros and cons with your physician before deciding on treatment.

For More Information:

Hysterectomy Educational Resources and Services Foundation
422 Bryn Mawr Avenue
Bala Cynwyd, PA 19004
(610) 667-7757

American Board of Obstetrics and Gynecology
2915 Vine Street
Dallas, TX 75204-1069
(214) 871-1619

Impotence

Sooner or later, it happens to almost *every* man. Still, most men don't like to talk about impotence—a chronic problem in achieving and maintaining an erection long enough to experience intercourse.

But impotence is nothing to feel ashamed of or humiliated about. As an inevitable—and normal—part of the aging process, the speed of a man's sexual response slows and the intensity of orgasm declines in response to a drop in testosterone levels, as well as to a decrease in blood circulation. In addition to reducing the need or desire to reach orgasm, this drop in hormone levels can result in the production of a smaller amount of semen during ejaculation. Don't think of these changes—which usually begin to occur in the late forties—as problems. Consider the benefit: You may find that you can enjoy intercourse longer before ejaculation.

And even if you do experience impotence rather than a

gradual decline of sexual function associated with aging, you can rest assured that you are not alone. It is estimated that more than 10 to 20 million American men are chronically impotent, including a quarter of men over age 65 and more than half of all men over 75.

Roughly three-fourths of all erection problems have at least some physical cause. To achieve an erection, there must be cooperation among blood vessels, nerves, and tissues. A number of health problems—including diabetes, heart and circulation problems, stroke, epilepsy, Alzheimer's disease, neurological disorders, alcohol and drug abuse, Parkinson's disease, and liver and kidney disease—can cause impotence. So can certain medications, including tranquilizers, diuretics, and anti-ulcer, antipsychotic, antidepressant, and antihypertensive drugs. Some over-the-counter antihistamines and decongestants can cause temporary impotence.

Other cases of impotence stem from psychological factors, such as relationship problems, stress, anxiety, grief, depression, fatigue, boredom, and guilt. Sexual intimacy can make some people feel very vulnerable, causing a number of stresses and uncomfortable feelings. With patience and treatment, most cases of psychological—as well as physical—impotence can be managed and overcome. Many natural remedies can also help.

Conventional Care

When it comes to impotence, a doctor's first task is to rule out a physical cause of the problem. This is usually done by a series of tests to assess the blood flow to the penis, the condition of the spinal cord, and testosterone and blood glucose levels. The doctor may recommend an at-home sleep test to find out if you experience erections during sleep. (If you have no erections during sleep, then there is probably a physical cause for the problem; if you do experience erections at night but not when you are with a partner, the cause is probably psychological.) In addition, your doctor will probably review any drugs you are taking, since impotence is a common side effect of many medications.

If your hormone levels fall below normal levels, testosterone shots or supplements may be prescribed. If you have inadequate blood flow to the penis, surgery may be required to open or unblock the arteries to the penis. And if all else fails, you may consider suction-pump devices, penile implants, or erection-producing medications.

The Natural Approach

If you suffer from impotence, first consult your doctor to see if you have an underlying organic or physical condition. Then try the natural remedies listed below. All of them can be used to supplement conventional medical treatment.

Herbal Medicine

Use one or more of the remedies listed below. For information on herbal medicine, see Chapter 2. Commercial preparations are also available; follow package directions.

- Ginkgo *(Ginkgo biloba):* This herb helps improve blood flow to the penis, which can help combat impotence. Ginkgo is usually available only in commercial preparations; follow package directions.
- Ginseng *(Panax quinquefolius):* This herb has long been considered a mild aphrodisiac. Ginseng preparations are widely available in health food stores; follow package directions.
- Yohimbine: This herb is the primary ingredient in a prescription drug used to treat impotence by increasing blood flow. It is commercially available, often in so-called "male potency formulas." Follow package directions.

Diet and Nutrition Supplements

Use one or more of the remedies listed below. For information on nutrition supplements and good food sources of particular nutrients, see Chapter 3.

- Vitamin A: The body needs vitamin A to produce the sex hormones that are essential for sexual function. Eat orange vegetables and other foods rich in beta-carotene (which the body converts to vitamin A). Also take a multivitamin, which should provide an adequate amount of this important vitamin.
- Vitamin C: This vitamin improves sperm mobility and helps keep the sperm from clumping together. Take up to 3,000 milligrams a day, in divided doses.
- Zinc: Prostate gland function and overall reproductive health depend on adequate intake of zinc. Take 15 to 50 milligrams a day.

Homeopathy

Use one homeopathic treatment at a time, based on your specific symptoms. For information on homeopathy, see Chapter 4. For dosage information, see pages 56–57. Discontinue use if the symptoms disappear.

- Agnus *(Agnus castus)* 30c: Use when intercourse has been frequent, but the erection is suddenly not firm enough for penetration. One dose twice daily, for up to five days.
- Conium *(Conium maculatum)* 30c: Use when there has been a long period without intercourse and there is desire, but the erection does not last. One dose twice daily, for up to five days.
- Ignatia *(Ignatia amara)* 30c: Use when distracted by grief or stress in other relationships. One dose twice daily, for up to five days.
- Lycopodium *(Lycopodium clavatum)* 30c: Use when the man would like to have intercourse but fears failure. One dose twice daily, for up to five days.

Acupressure

Use one or more of the acupressure points listed below. For information on acupressure, see Chapter 5. For diagrams showing the specific pressure points, see pages 88–91.

- Bladder 23: Two finger-widths away from the spine at waist level (in line with the belly button).
- Conception Vessel 6: Three finger-widths below the belly button.
- Kidney 1: At the base of the ball of the foot, in the middle of the sole.
- Kidney 3: Inside the ankle, in the depression between the back of the ankle and the Achilles tendon.
- Spleen 12: In the center of the crease where the leg joins the trunk.

An Ounce of Prevention

Being in good physical condition can improve potency as well as overall health. Eat a well-balanced diet, and get regular exercise. Avoid alcohol, which can cause temporary impotence, as well as smoking, which restricts blood flow throughout the body. When making love, take your time, relax, and enjoy some foreplay. Have intercourse more often, since testosterone levels remain higher in men who have sex more frequently.

If natural remedies don't help and your doctor can't find a physical basis for the problem, contact a psychologist or mental health professional. Statistics indicate that therapy can help in four out of five cases of psychologically based impotence.

Warning Signs

Impotence shows up at the least convenient times—and with no warning or invitation. A single episode should not be cause for alarm, but a pattern of difficulty maintaining an erection merits a discussion with a medical professional to rule out physical problems.

For More Information:

Potency Restored
8630 Fenton Street, Suite 218
Silver Spring, MD 20910
(301) 588-5777

Impotence Institute of America
10400 Little Patuxent Parkway, Suite 485
Columbia, MD 21044
(410) 715-9605

American Association of Sex Educators, Counselors and Therapists
435 North Michigan Avenue, Suite 1717
Chicago, IL 60611
(312) 644-0828

Impotence Information Center
American Medical Systems
Minneapolis, MN 55440
(800) 543-9632

Incontinence

Urinary incontinence (or loss of bladder control) can be embarrassing—even humiliating—but many people understand the problem because they experience it themselves. More than 10 million people—including at least 10 to 20 percent of all older adults—live with incontinence, though most won't talk about it much.

Before age 65, incontinence affects three to fives times more women than men. Women who have had children experience more problems because pregnancy places intense pressure on the bladder and muscles of the pelvic floor; in addition, labor and delivery can tear the muscles and surrounding tissues, sometimes leaving them less resilient than before. About 40 percent of women experience some incontinence during pregnancy, and 10 percent continue to have problems afterward. At menopause the decrease in estrogen can weaken the pelvic floor muscles and thin the lining of the urethra, loosening the seal at the neck of the bladder.

Men experience less incontinence, in part because they have longer urethras (10 inches, versus about 2 inches for women). The prostate gland also helps support a man's urethra, helping to prevent leakage. An enlarged prostate, however, can put pressure on the bladder, so that after age 65 men and women have an almost equal chance of becoming incontinent.

Still, you don't have to accept incontinence as an inevitable part of aging. Most causes of incontinence can be either controlled or cured. Incontinence isn't a disease but a symptom of an underlying problem, such as weak muscles in the pelvic floor or an obstruction of the bladder outflow.

There are five basic types of chronic incontinence:

- Stress incontinence is a condition in which small amounts of urine dribble out when you exercise, cough, laugh, sneeze, or move in other ways that put pressure on the bladder. Most cases of stress incontinence are associated with weak muscles in the pelvic floor, though in severe cases there may be nerve damage or tears in the sphincter muscles.
- Urge incontinence usually involves the loss of large amounts or urine with little warning. It occurs when the need to urinate comes on so quickly that there isn't enough time to make it to the toilet. Urge incontinence can be caused by stroke, Parkinson's disease, kidney or bladder stones, or bladder infection.
- Overflow incontinence involves urination with no warning or sensation. In such cases the urine overflows and spills out when a person shifts position or stands up. Often the person feels the need to urinate again a few minutes later but cannot empty the bladder completely. People with overflow incontinence have a high risk of bladder infection. It sometimes occurs following pelvic surgery or a bladder suspension operation. Diabetes or an enlarged prostate can contribute to overflow incontinence as well.

- Reflex incontinence involves involuntary, spontaneous urination—no warnings, no urges, no rush to the bathroom. This lack of bladder control is usually caused by spinal cord injury, diabetes, multiple sclerosis, and other serious medical conditions.
- Functional incontinence strikes people who have normal bladder control and warnings but cannot reach the bathroom fast enough due to physical limitations.

In addition, temporary incontinence can be caused by the use of diuretics and other medications. Most cases of incontinence can be controlled or managed by correcting the underlying health problem or condition.

More than half of all people with incontinence fail to seek help for the problem, though experts estimate that more than 80 percent of them could be cured or significantly helped. A number of treatments, including the following natural remedies, can assist with restoring bladder control.

Conventional Care

Though many people find incontinence difficult to discuss openly with a doctor, there are things a doctor may be able to do to help the condition. For one thing, diagnostic tests should be done to rule out infection or early signs of diabetes or heart disease.

Most doctors will recommend the Kegel exercises (see the box on page 331). Some also may recommend electrical stimulation of the pelvic floor or even surgery to tighten up the tissue. Be sure to mention any prescription or over-the-counter drugs you have been taking, since some can change urinary function or cause incontinence.

Some doctors will recommend the use of a pessary, a silicone or rubber device that fits into the top of the vagina in much the same way that a diaphragm does. The pessary physically raises the bladder to a more normal position, reducing the likelihood of leakage due to stress incontinence.

Estrogen replacement therapy may also help. Certain drugs can ease urge incontinence by relaxing the bladder and keeping it from contracting. Injections of collagen around the sphincter can tighten the seal and prevent leakage; surgery on the bladder neck is recommended in severe cases.

Words of Wisdom

"Kegels do help some people—I certainly wouldn't discourage anyone from doing them—but sometimes muscle tone isn't the cause of the incontinence. There may be a low-grade or chronic infection that has not been resolved, or the tissue may have been damaged by the trauma of childbirth. Homeopathy is particularly helpful in these cases because it not only treats the incontinence, it also addresses the cause of the incontinence."

Eleanor Herschberger, N.D.
Tallmadge, Ohio

The Natural Approach

All of the natural remedies listed below can be used to supplement conventional medical treatment.

Herbal Medicine

Use one or more of the remedies listed below. For information on herbal medicine, see Chapter 2. Commercial preparations are also available; follow package directions.

- Cypress *(Cupressus sempervirens):* Cypress oil helps reduce excess fluid production. Add 50 drops of the oil to 5 teaspoons of almond oil, and massage into the lower abdomen twice a day.
- Huang qi *(Astragalus membranaceus):* This herb helps regulate the metabolism of water. Commercially pre-

pared capsules and tinctures are available; follow
package directions.

Foods to Avoid

Avoid coffee, tea, and other drinks that contain caffeine, which tends to
overstimulate the bladder. Do not, however, limit overall fluid intake; you
need to drink at least eight 8-ounce glasses of water—one full gallon—
every day for your body to work at its best.

Homeopathy

Use one homeopathic treatment at a time, based on your
specific symptoms. For information on homeopathy, see
Chapter 2. For dosage information, see pages 56–57. Discontinue use if the symptoms disappear.

- Causticum *(Causticum Hahnemanni)* 6c: Use when
  urine leakage occurs as a result of coughing, sneezing,
  nose blowing, or other outbursts. One dose four times
  a day, for up to three weeks.
- Ferrum phos. *(Ferrum phosphoricum)* 6c: Use when
  urinary incontinence is accompanied by bladder pain
  and the frequent urge to urinate. One dose four times
  a day, for up to three days.
- Nux *(Strychnos nux vomica)* 6c: Use when there are
  involuntary dribbles of urine. One dose four times a
  day, for up to three days.
- Pulsatilla *(Pulsatilla nigricans)* 6c: Use when urine
  leaks when you sit down, walk, or pass gas. One dose
  every four hours, for up to one week.

Acupressure

Use one or more of the acupressure points listed below.
For information on acupressure, see Chapter 5. For diagrams showing the specific pressure points, see pages 88–
91.

- Bladder 28: In the lower back, two finger-widths on either side of the sacrum.
- Conception Vessel 6: Two finger-widths below the navel, on the midline of the abdomen.
- Kidney 3: On the inside of the ankle, in the hollow halfway between the anklebone and the back of the ankle, level with the anklebone.
- Spleen 6: On the inside of the leg, four finger-widths above the tip of the anklebone and just inside the bone of the leg.

An Ounce of Prevention

Many people with incontinence simply have lost the muscle tone in their pelvic floor, which supports the bladder, uterus, and other internal organs. The easiest way to deal with this problem is to strengthen the muscles by doing the Kegel exercises listed in the box on page 331.

Extra pounds can also cause the pelvic floor to sag, giving you yet another good reason to shed the extra weight. (See Chapter 8 for information on weight loss.) Incontinence provides yet another motivation to quit smoking— the nicotine in cigarettes irritates the bladder, and a smoker's cough can cause problems with stress incontinence.

While waiting for these lifestyle changes to take effect, try the technique known as "double voiding." Empty your bladder, then relax a minute and try again. You might also try urinating, then standing up for a minute, sitting down and leaning forward, then trying again.

Warning Signs

If you develop urinary incontinence, you'll know it. The most common symptoms include the urgent and frequent need for urination; bed-wetting; and leakage during episodes of physical stress, such as coughing, sneezing, or laughing. Sometimes incontinence is caused by a urinary tract infection, which should be treated with antibiotics. If you feel pain or burning when you urinate, in addition to experiencing incontinence, contact your doctor to find out if you have an infection.

For More Information:

National Association for Continence
P.O. Box 8310
Spartanburg, SC 29305-8310
(800) BLADDER
(803) 579-7900

Simon Foundation for Continence
P.O. Box 815
Wilmette, IL 60091
(708) 864-3913

Kegel Exercises: Give Your Bladder a Workout

The bladder is a muscular tank able to hold 8 to 16 ounces of urine. But like any other muscles, those involved with bladder control must be in good shape to work their best. That's where Kegel exercises come in.

Kegel exercises, named for Dr. Arnold Kegel, the gynecologist who popularized them, can help cure or improve stress incontinence by toning and strengthening the pelvic floor and the muscles that control the flow of urine. To exercise your bladder, follow these steps:

- Locate the appropriate muscles by repeatedly stopping your urine in midstream. The muscles you squeeze around your urethra and anus to stop the urine are the muscles you want to work on.
- Practice squeezing and releasing these muscles several times each time you urinate. Once you are familiar with them, practice squeezing them when you are not urinating. (Tip: If your abdomen or buttocks move, you are not using the right muscles.)
- During each exercise contraction, hold the squeeze for three seconds, then relax for three seconds. Repeat this 10 to 15 times per session, three or four sessions a day.

Kegel exercises are easy to do and remarkably effective. Try doing them while waiting at red lights, talking on the phone, or watching television. If you do them properly, no one will know you are doing them except you.

Insomnia

Insomnia can be a nightmare, especially for older people. You're desperate for sleep, but it seems that the more exhausted you feel, the harder it is to rest.

As we get older, we awaken more often than we used to, and we spend more time fully awake in the middle of the night. Sleep studies have found that by age 65, most people wake up at least a dozen times a night and spend only about half an hour in the most restful periods of deep sleep. (A 20-year-old, in comparison, snoozes virtually without waking and accumulates about two hours of high-quality, deep sleep.)

But these changes in sleep patterns do not necessarily reflect a sleep problem. Insomnia refers to any of three sleep disorders: difficulty falling asleep (more than 45 minutes); early morning awakening; or frequent night awakenings (six or more a night). You have insomnia, however, only if you experience these symptoms and they leave you feeling tired and worn down. After all, you are the ultimate judge of how much pillow time your body needs.

Sooner or later almost everyone experiences insomnia. In fact, during the course of a year, nearly one out of every three people suffers from the problem at least once. Short-term insomnia—sleeplessness that lasts a few nights to a few weeks—usually stems from worry or concern about a stressful situation. Long-term insomnia—sleeplessness lasting months or years—often comes from general anxiety, medication, chronic pain, depression, hypoglycemia, apnea, or other physical disorders.

Conventional Care

To determine the cause of your sleeplessness, start by reviewing all the prescription and nonprescription medications you're taking to find out if any could be contributing to the problem. Pain relievers, cold remedies, appetite suppressants, and decongestants, and medications for asthma, hypertension, heart disease, and thyroid problems can all interfere with a good night's sleep.

Your doctor will probably make several other suggestions, such as the following:

- Save your bed for sleeping and sex; don't eat, watch TV, or read in it.
- Make sure your bedroom is dark, quiet, and well ventilated.
- Don't nap during the day.
- Don't be a slave to the clock; go to bed when you feel tired, not when you think you should sleep.
- Don't lie around; get out of bed anytime you lie awake for more than 15 minutes.
- Wake up at the same time each day, even if you feel sleepy.

In some cases, your doctor may prescribe drugs to promote sleep. Each year four to six million Americans have prescriptions filled for sleep-inducing sedatives. Never take sleeping pills for more than two weeks; while they help bring on sleep, they actually interfere with deep sleep. In addition, they can cause a "hangover" effect, which is especially dangerous in older people. Studies have found that older people taking long-acting sleeping pills are 70 percent more likely to fall and fracture a hip than those not taking sleeping pills.

If your doctor suspects a physical cause of your insomnia, you may be referred to a sleep specialist, who will monitor your sleep patterns and brain-wave patterns during the night. If psychological stress contributes to the problem, you may be referred to a psychologist or psychiatrist to explore other issues related to the problem.

Words of Wisdom

"There are two kinds of insomnia—one is when people can't go to sleep, and the other is when they can't stay asleep. People who wake up in the middle of the night often experience hypoglycemia or low blood sugar. What they need to do is to take some kind of carbohydrate snack before they go to bed. A nice choice might be some warm milk with honey, maybe with a graham cracker."

Don Canavan, N.D.
Albany, California

The Natural Approach

In addition to the remedies suggested below, experiment with deep breathing and relaxation exercises in bed while you are trying to fall asleep. Concentrate on breathing deeply into your belly to reduce tension and stress. (For more information, see Chapter 9.) All of the natural remedies listed below can be used to supplement conventional medical treatment.

Herbal Medicine

Use one or more of the remedies listed below. For information on herbal medicine, see Chapter 2. Commercial preparations are also available; follow package directions.

- California poppy *(Eschscholzia californica):* This herb has gentle, nonaddictive tranquilizing properties. Commercially prepared tinctures are available; follow package directions.
- Hops *(Humulus lupulus):* This herb has a sedative effect. To make an infusion, use 2 teaspoons of herb per cup of boiling water and steep for 5 minutes; strain, and drink one cup before bedtime. Commercially prepared tinctures are available; follow package directions.
- Passionflower *(Passiflora incarnata):* This herb calms the nervous system and promotes sleep. To prepare passionflower tea, use 2 to 3 teaspoons of dried herb per cup of boiling water; steep for 5 minutes, strain, and drink a cup before bed. Commercially prepared tinctures are available; follow package directions.
- Valerian *(Valeriana officinalis):* This herb contains chemicals, known as valepotriates, that have sedative properties. To prepare an infusion, use 2 teaspoons of powdered herb per cup of water; steep for 10 minutes. Strain, and drink one cup before bed.

Diet and Nutrition Supplements

Use one or more of the remedies listed below. For information on nutrition supplements and good food sources of particular nutrients, see Chapter 3.

- Calcium and magnesium: A deficiency in calcium and magnesium can cause you to wake up after a few hours of sleep and have trouble getting back to sleep. Take 1,500 milligrams of calcium and 750 milligrams of magnesium a day.
- Melatonin: During sleep the pineal gland in the brain secretes the hormone melatonin, which helps regulate

the body's sleep-wake cycle. Melatonin levels drop as we get older, so a supplement may help induce sleep. Supplements are commercially available; follow package directions.

• Tryptophan foods: Before bed, snack on foods high in sleep-producing tryptophan, such as turkey, bananas, figs, dates, yogurt, milk, tuna, whole-grain crackers, and peanut butter.

Foods to Avoid

Foods that contain tyramines cause the brain to release norepinephrine, a stimulant. In the evening before bed, pass on tyramine-rich foods, including caffeine, alcohol, sugar, tobacco, cheese, chocolate, sauerkraut, wine, bacon, ham, sausage, eggplant, potatoes, spinach, and tomatoes.

Homeopathy

Use one homeopathic treatment at a time, based on your specific symptoms. For information on homeopathy, see Chapter 4. For dosage information, see pages 56–57. Discontinue use if the symptoms disappear.

• Aconite. *(Aconitum napellus)* 30c: Use if nightmares, particularly about death, accompany sleep problems. One dose 1 hour before bed, for one week. Repeat if you wake up and can't get back to sleep.
• Coffea *(Coffea cruda)* 30 c: Use if your mind is active and you toss and turn all night. One dose 1 hour before bed, for one week. Repeat if you wake up and can't get back to sleep.
• Ignatia *(Ignatia amara)* 30c: Use if you are fearful of bedtime, possibly due to nightmares. One dose 1 hour before bed, for one week. Repeat if you wake up and can't get back to sleep.
• Nux *(Strychnos nux vomica)* 30c: Use if you fall asleep but wake up at 3 A.M. or so and remain awake, perhaps falling asleep again just before morning. One

dose 1 hour before bed, for one week. Repeat if you wake up with nightmares and can't get back to sleep.

Acupressure

Use one or more of the acupressure points listed below. For information on acupressure, see Chapter 5. For diagrams showing the specific pressure points, see pages 88–91.

- Bladder 62: In the first indentation directly below the outer anklebone.
- Gallbladder 12: Behind the ears, in the hollow under the bone.
- Heart 7: On the inside of the wrist crease, in the hollow level with the little finger.
- Kidney 6: Directly below the inside of the anklebone, in a slight indentation.

An Ounce of Prevention

To prevent insomnia, get regular exercise, but avoid strenuous exercise within two hours before bedtime. Avoid smoking or consuming caffeine or alcohol for three or four hours before bedtime. That before-bed nightcap might make you feel sleepy at first, but it will make you more likely to awaken during the night. Sex is a natural relaxant; under the right circumstances, intercourse can help you unwind and enjoy a good night's sleep.

If you tend to awaken in the middle of the night, your blood-sugar levels may be falling too low. To avoid the problem, try having a high-carbohydrate snack before bed. Milk, whole-grain crackers, peanut butter, and bananas are particularly good choices because they contain the sleep-inducing chemical tryptophan, in addition to being good sources of carbohydrates, which can help your body maintain a moderate blood-sugar levels into the night.

Warning Signs

If you have insomnia, you'll recognize it by the sleepy feeling during the day and the restless feeling at night. In addition to sleepless nights, you will almost certainly experience trouble concentrating and daytime fatigue and irritability. When you're functioning with a sleep deficit, you may also notice that your reflexes have grown sluggish, and you may be more prone to illness, since the body needs sleep to keep the immune system working its best.

Fortunately it's relatively easy for the body to "catch up" on sleep. A single night of full sleep—one in which you sleep until you naturally awaken—will allow you to regain about 90 percent of the mental sharpness you lost due to sleep deprivation. Add a second full night, and you should be as sharp as ever.

For More Information:

American Sleep Disorder Institute
1610 14th Street, N.W., Suite 300
Rochester, MN 55901
(507) 287-6006

Better Sleep Council
333 Commerce Street
Alexandria, VA 22314
(703) 683-8371

National Sleep Foundation
1367 Connecticut Avenue, N.W., Suite 200
Washington, DC 20036
(202) 785-2300

Beyond Snoring: Sleep Apnea

In an ideal world we would all awaken from sleep feeling refreshed and well rested. But as every sleep-deprived person knows, this is not always the case. The problem can be particularly severe for the 20 million Americans who suffer from sleep apnea.

Apnea is a common problem that causes sleepers to stop breathing for periods of ten seconds or more—as many as three hundred times a night. It usually occurs in deep sleep, when the muscles in the throat relax, allowing the pharynx to collapse and block the airway. After a few seconds without breathing, the body sends a signal to the brain that it is low on oxygen, and an automatic reflex kicks in, reminding the body to begin breathing again, often with an explosive grunt or gasp. Because their sleep is constantly interrupted, people with apnea often feel sleepy during the day, even if they spend long hours in bed "asleep."

Sleep experts estimate that about half of chronic snorers over age 40 have apnea.

People with apnea should consult a doctor because the problem can cause serious health problems, including high blood pressure, enlargement of the heart, and increased risk of stroke. Each year, two to three thousand people with apnea die of cardiac arrest in the night.

If you suffer from apnea, avoid sleeping pills and alcohol, which can induce a deeper sleep and exacerbate apnea. Also, try sleeping on your side. You might consider attaching a sock with a tennis ball to the back of your pajamas or nightgown to prevent you from rolling over onto your back. People who are overweight tend to suffer from apnea more often than slender sleepers, giving you another good reason to shed those extra pounds.

Menopause

Menopause can be a welcome spring shower—or a violent thunderstorm with gale-force winds. Some women glide through menopause with nary a symptom or complaint, while others must endure a number of difficult physical and psychological adjustments as they work their way through the "change of life."

At the most basic level, menopause is nothing more than the cessation of ovulation and menstrual cycles. It usually occurs in women between the ages of 45 and 55, with the average age being 51. Most women experience irregular periods for five to seven years before their cycle stops entirely. (This erratic time is known as perimenopause.) A woman is considered to have passed through menopause after going one full year without menstrual periods.

Menopausal symptoms—including hot flashes, vaginal dryness, and anxiety—occur in response to changes in estrogen and progesterone levels in the body. (For information on vaginal dryness, see page 387; for information on anxiety, see page 159.) Hot flashes occur when estrogen levels drop, causing a sudden adjustment in the body's thermostat and an abrupt "flash" of heat. (The pituitary gland in the brain controls both estrogen levels and body temperature; hence the link between hormones and heat.)

Typically, the heat of a hot flash begins in the chest and spreads to the neck, face, and arms. It can be accompanied by sweating and heart palpitations, and it may be followed by chills. Three out of every four menopausal women experience hot flashes, which can occur as often as once an hour and can last for three or four minutes at a stretch. For most women, hot flashes are mild and end within two years, but 25 percent of women who experience hot flashes suffer from them for more than five years, and about 10 percent "flash" for the rest of their lives.

In addition to the physical changes, many women experience mood swings, depression, insomnia, and irritability during menopause. These psychological disturbances can be caused by organic changes and shifting hormone levels, but they can also be exacerbated by the other life changes taking place during the late forties and early fifties, such as children leaving home and career-related stresses.

The discomforts of menopause can be especially severe if menstruation stops abruptly, either naturally or following the surgical removal of the ovaries. Whatever the trigger event, natural remedies can be very useful in treating symptoms of menopause.

Conventional Care

When women suffer from the uncomfortable symptoms of menopause, most doctors recommend estrogen replacement therapy, which can provide relief in women who are good candidates for treatment. (See the box on estrogen replacement treatment on pages 347–349.)

Words of Wisdom

"One important herb that can really make a difference in a woman's life when she is going through menopause is evening primrose oil. This herb encourages hormonal balance in the body, which is especially important when estrogen levels are dropping. The primrose oil helps with hot flashes and mood changes. For some women, menopause can be difficult, but with this herb, menopause is just another part of life."

Phoebe Reeve, M.A.
Member of the American Herbalists Guild
Annandale, Virginia

The Natural Approach

All of the natural remedies listed below can be used to supplement conventional medical treatment.

Herbal Medicine

Use one or more of the remedies listed below. For information on herbal medicine, see Chapter 2. Commercial preparations are also available; follow package directions.

- Black cohosh *(Cimicifuga racemosa):* This herb has long been used to manage menstrual and menopausal complaints due to its estrogenic effects, meaning it acts like the female hormone estrogen. For a decoction, boil ½ teaspoon of powdered root per cup of water for 30 minutes. Strain, and drink 2 tablespoons every few hours, up to one cup per day.
- Dandelion *(Taraxacum officinale):* This plant has mild diuretic effects, which can help to relieve menopausal water retention. Dandelions can be eaten fresh in sal-

ads. Dandelion tea and capsules are available at health food stores; follow package instructions.

- Fenugreek *(Trigonella foenum-graecum):* Fenugreek seeds contain diosgenin, a chemical similar to the female hormone estrogen. The herb is often used in the treatment of hot flashes and depression associated with menopause. Fenugreek tea is available at health food stores. To prepare a decoction, boil 2 teaspoons of seeds in 1 cup of water. Simmer for 10 minutes; strain, and drink up to three cups a day.

- Licorice *(Glycyrrhiza glabra):* This herb is often used to treat the complaints of menopause because it contains glycyrrhizin, a hormonelike compound that helps stabilize hormone levels. Commercial preparations are available in health food stores; follow package directions.

- Primrose oil: Hot flashes often respond well to primrose oil, which acts as a sedative and diuretic. Commercial products are available; follow package directions.

- Wild yam *(D. villosa):* This herb contains plant hormones very similar to the female hormone progesterone. In fact, until 1970, this plant was used in the manufacture of birth control pills. This herb is commercially available from health food stores.

Diet and Nutrition Supplements

Use one or more of the remedies listed below. For information on nutrition supplements and good food sources of particular nutrients, see Chapter 3.

- Calcium and magnesium: Osteoporosis, or thinning of the bones, often begins at menopause when estrogen levels drop. To help prevent this dangerous side effect of menopause, take 1,500 milligrams of calcium and 750 milligrams of magnesium a day. (For more information on osteoporosis, see page 358.)

- Soy: Soybeans and other foods rich in soy protein contain phytoestrogens, or molecules very similar to estrogen and progesterone. A menopausal woman who eats lots of soy protein can retain the benefits she had previously received from her body's natural estrogen. Try to consume 25 grams of soy daily; a soy burger contains about 18 grams, a glass of soy milk about 8 grams. Powdered soy supplements are also available at health food stores.

- Vitamin E: This vitamin helps combat vaginal dryness, control hot flashes, and increase the production of hormones. Take 400 to 800 IU a day.

Foods to Avoid

Hot flashes can be exacerbated by alcohol (which opens the blood vessels) and caffeine (which is a stimulant). To minimize hot flashes, avoid both alcohol and caffeine.

Homeopathy

Use one homeopathic treatment at a time, based on your specific symptoms. For information on homeopathy, see Chapter 4. For dosage information, see pages 56–57. Discontinue use if the symptoms disappear.

- Amyl nit. *(Amyl nitrite)* 30c: Use when hot flashes accompany menopause. One dose twice daily, for one week.
- Bryonia *(Bryonia alba)* 30c: Use when menopause is accompanied by vaginal dryness and constipation. One dose twice a day for one week.
- Calcarea *(Calcarea carbonica)* 30c: Use when weight gain, phobias, panic attacks, backache, and hot flashes accompany menopause. One dose twice a day, for up to one week.
- Lachesis *(Trigonocephalus lachesis)* 30c: Use when menopause is accompanied by headaches or migraines, dizziness, insomnia, hot flashes, verbosity,

and excitability. One dose twice a day, for up to one week.

- Pulsatilla *(Pulsatilla nigricans)* 30c: Use when menopause is accompanied by hot flashes, hemorrhoids, varicose veins, and weepiness. One dose twice a day, for one week.
- Sepia *(Sepia officinalis)* 30c: Use when menopause is accompanied by vaginal dryness, hot flashes, chills, irritability, and an aversion to sexual intercourse. One dose twice a day, for up to one week.

The Menopause Workout

One important ingredient in the treatment of menopause that is far too often overlooked is regular aerobic exercise, which can help to counteract both the physical and psychological difficulties associated with menopause. (For more information on aerobic exercise, see pages 97–100.)

Acupressure

Use one or more of the acupressure points listed below. For information on acupressure, see Chapter 5. For diagrams showing the specific pressure points, see pages 88–91.

- Conception Vessel 17: Three thumb-widths up from the center of the base of the breastbone.
- Kidney 1: On the sole of the foot, in the depression just below the ball of the foot, between the two foot pads.
- Large Intestine 4: In the webbing between the thumb and the index finger, at the end of the crease made when the thumb and index finger are pressed together.
- Spleen 6: Four finger-widths above the tip of the anklebone, in the middle of the inside of the leg.
- Triple Warmer 5: On the outside of the forearm, three

finger-widths above the wrist, in the depression between the arm bones.

An Ounce of Prevention

Menopause is a natural—and inevitable—part of the aging
process. It is an important stage of a woman's reproductive
cycle and need not be feared or met with apprehension.

Warning Signs

One out of every two women experiences some symptoms
associated with menopause, and about one in four finds
those symptoms uncomfortable to distressing. While some
women experience increased energy and enthusiasm for
life during menopause, most women complain of certain
common symptoms including:

- Hot flashes and sweating
- Facial flushing
- Vaginal dryness
- Headaches
- Heart palpitations
- Irregular periods
- Joint pain
- Depression
- Anxiety
- Irritability
- Lack of concentration
- Mood swings
- Sleep disturbances
- Forgetfulness

For More Information:

American Menopause Foundation
Madison Square Station
P.O. Box 2013
New York, NY 10010
(212) 475-3107

North American Menopause Society
c/o University Hospitals of Cleveland
Dept. OB/GYN
Room 7024
1110 Euclid Avenue
Cleveland, OH 44106
(216) 844-8748

Society for Menstrual Cycle Research
10559 North 104th Place
Scottsdale, AZ 85258
(602) 451-9731

The Estrogen Question

It's a tough question: After menopause, should you take supplemental estrogen or not? It's a trade-off: Estrogen replacement therapy (ERT) will lower your risk of developing certain health problems, but it may increase the risk of others.

In the past doctors prescribed ERT primarily to relieve menopausal complaints. Today ERT is often prescribed for its potentially life-saving health benefits. But ERT is not right for every woman. Your answer to the Estrogen Question should be based on an assessment of your individual risks and family medical history. Consider the following:

THE PROS

Estrogen protects against heart disease. Heart disease and stroke
   kill more than half of all women over age 50, more than all forms of
   cancer combined. ERT lowers the risk of heart disease by about 50

percent by reducing levels of low-density lipoprotein cholesterol (the "bad" cholesterol) and increasing levels of high-density lipoprotein cholesterol (the "good" cholesterol). Simply being postmenopausal puts a woman at higher risk for heart disease. If she has just one additional risk factor—if she smokes, has high blood pressure, HDL cholesterol below 35, diabetes, or a family history of heart disease—she is at high risk for cardiovascular disease and would most likely benefit from hormone therapy.

- **Estrogen helps prevent osteoporosis.** ERT lowers the risk of developing osteoporosis by slowing the rate of bone loss after menopause. Studies show that estrogen therapy can reduce the risk of osteoporosis fractures by up to 60 percent.
- **ERT may reduce your risk of developing Alzheimer's disease.** A recent study found that the longer a woman took estrogen, the lower her odds of getting Alzheimer's disease. For women who took ERT for 10 years, the risk dropped by 30 to 40 percent.
- **Hormone therapy can ease common menopausal complaints.** ERT can relieve hot flashes, vaginal dryness, mood swings, and other menopausal symptoms related to a drop in estrogen.

The Cons

Some studies suggest that ERT may increase a woman's risk of breast cancer. There is conflicting evidence about the link between ERT and breast cancer. While some studies show an increased cancer risk, others indicate that low doses of estrogen taken for less than five years do not increase breast cancer rates at all. To make matters more confusing, recent research by the American Cancer Society has shown that women who take ERT may be less likely to die from breast cancer, even if they are more likely to develop the disease. The study found that women who reported using estrogen for up to ten years had a 16 percent lower risk of dying from breast cancer, and those who began using estrogen before they were 40 were 34 percent less likely to die from the disease. Researchers speculate that ERT may encourage the growth of slow-growing tumors and suppress the more aggressive (and more deadly) ones. Still, women at high risk of developing breast cancer may want to avoid additional estrogen, and all women taking estrogen should make a point to have an annual mammogram. (Talk to your doctor about the benefits of ERT and heart disease in comparison with the risks of ERT and breast cancer; researchers estimate that for each additional breast cancer death caused by hormone therapy, eight other deaths from heart disease would be prevented.)

- **Estrogen may raise a woman's risk of developing endometrial cancer.** Studies suggest that ERT increases the risk of developing endometrial cancer (cancer of the lining of the uterus). Combining estrogen and progestin (a synthetic form of the hormone progesterone) offsets the risk, but the addition of the progesterone reduces the cholesterol-reducing benefits of the estrogen.
- **ERT may make fibroids worse.** Estrogen can increase the size of fibroids (benign tumors in the uterus), causing bleeding and pain. Without supplemental estrogen, most fibroids shrink after menopause.
- **Hormone therapy can cause gallstones.** Studies suggest that ERT more than doubles a woman's chances of developing gallstones.
- **Some women don't like the side effects of ERT.** Hormone therapy can cause a number of unpleasant side effects, including hormone-related weight gain, fluid retention, nausea, headaches, breast tenderness, and regular monthly bleeding. More serious side effects—which should be treated by a doctor—include persistent headaches, swelling, and the formation of blood clots.

The raging hormone debate leaves many women baffled about what to do. Only one out of every four women over 50 takes supplemental estrogen, and 60 percent of those who start on ERT stop within twelve months. Most women quit ERT because they don't like the side effects. Unfortunately, ERT's protective effects disappear once a woman stops taking hormones.

ERT can be administered as a pill, vaginal cream, or skin patch. Before starting ERT, a woman should have a complete physical examination, including a breast exam and mammogram, a pelvic exam, a Pap smear, and blood tests for cholesterol, glucose, thyroid, and liver function.

A Word About Natural Hormones

You can have it all—the benefits of hormone replacement therapy—without the side effects caused by synthetic hormones. The solution: natural plant estrogen.

Plants contain phytoestrogens, or compounds that have molecules very similar to those of the human hormones estrogen and progesterone. In the body these plant estrogens offer many of the same healthful benefits that human estrogen does; they also boost the effectiveness of the body's own estrogen and help keep hormone levels on an even keel.

Natural plant estrogens are less powerful—and safer—than synthetic estrogens made by pharmaceutical companies. Consider the example of diethylstilbestrol (DES), a synthetic estrogen that doctors once prescribed routinely to regulate the menstrual cycle and to prevent premature labor (among other uses). On a molecular basis DES closely resembles a plant estrogen known as P-anol, but these two substances have dramatically different effects on the body. While the plant version has proved harmless in small quantities, DES has been shown to cause several types of cancer, including vaginal and cervical cancer in daughters and testicular cancer in sons of mothers who were given DES during pregnancy.

The DES story is not an anomaly. When used at appropriate doses (no more than the body would have produced before menopause), natural plant hormones have no known side effects. On the other hand, synthetic hormones have many, including migraine headaches, fluid retention, epilepsy, depression, and heart problems, among many others.

Natural plant hormone supplements can be administered topically (in the form of skin creams or oils), sublingually (as drops under the tongue), or orally (as capsules). They can also be consumed as foods or dietary supplements; soybeans and flaxseed oil are two common dietary sources of plant hormones, but more than three hundred other herbs also contain these compounds. Many natural hormone products are available commercially.

Most natural hormone creams are made from Mexican wild yams. These hormone-rich plants contain diosgenin, a substance that can be extracted and processed into a hormone that is molecularly identical to the progesterone produced in a woman's body. In fact, until 1970, wild yams were the sole source of the progesterone used in birth control pills.

Natural hormone creams are available in health food stores. Avoid plain Mexican yam products; they contain diosgenin, but the body cannot convert diosgenin into progesterone on its own. Instead, look for products containing processed or micronized progesterone.

When using hormone creams, choose a product containing 475 milligrams of progesterone per ounce. The cream should be applied to the breasts and buttocks daily, using about one ounce of cream every two weeks. It is also available in capsule form. (For specific dosage and usage information, follow package directions.)

Obesity

It's not easy being fat: Obesity takes both an emotional and a physical toll on all those who suffer from it. If you are more than 20 percent above the normal weight for your age, build, and height, you are considered obese. Those extra pounds also put you at greater risk of a number of health problems, including heart disease, diabetes, high blood pressure, stroke, gallbladder disease, hemorrhoids, varicose veins, and kidney and liver problems.

Dieting may be part of the American way of life, but experts estimate that 20 to 50 percent of all Americans remain obese, despite obsessing about what they put in their mouths. In most cases, overeating combined with a lack of exercise causes obesity, though genetics, glandular malfunctions, cultural background, and social and emotional factors also play a role. (For more information on diet, see Chapter 7; on exercise, see Chapter 6.)

Conventional Care

As any veteran of the battle of the bulge knows, obesity can be very difficult to control. While countless diet plans crowd bookstore shelves, when it comes to weight loss most physicians recommend a traditional diet restricting caloric intake to 1,500 calories a day and adding 15 to 20 minutes of aerobic exercise three to four times a week. Weight loss should be limited to one or two pounds a week; generally, the more gradually the weight comes off, the more likely it will stay off.

In some cases doctors will prescribe appetite suppressants, but they can have negative side effects, including nervousness, restlessness, sleeplessness, high blood pressure, drowsiness, and headache.

Surgical options include liposuction (in which an incision is made and fat is sucked out of the body), colectomy (in which part of the intestine is bypassed, limiting the length of the intestine in which food can be absorbed by the body), and stomach stapling (in which the size of the stomach is reduced, to limit physically the amount of food that can be consumed). All of these procedures have significant dangers, and they aren't guaranteed to work; after surgery many people lose weight, only to regain it later.

Regular exercise increases your metabolic rate. In fact, your body continues to burn calories for hours after you stop exercising. If you exercise regularly while losing weight, you tend to lose mostly fat, rather than fat and lean muscle mass.

Also, be sure not to skip meals. When you go hungry, your metabolic rate drops in order to conserve fuel. In fact, you can eat up to 20 percent more calories and maintain your weight if the calories are spread throughout the day, maintaining an even energy supply to the body. Crash diets, missed meals, and starvation confuse the body's appetite control system and metabolism. Your goal should be to provide a steady supply of nutritious foods for your body to use throughout the day.

Words of Wisdom

"The Chinese on average consume 20 percent more calories than we do in the United States, yet they are much less obese, even when we adjust for different levels of physical activity. It has to do with the macronutrient composition of the diet, and the balance between the carbohydrate, fat, and protein in the diet. In China they eat about 70 percent of their calories from carbohydrates, compared to 40 percent here. They get 10 to 15 percent of their calories from fat, compared to 35 to 40 percent here. The amount of protein is more or less the same—about 10 to 12 percent—but the source of protein is very different. In the United States 70 percent of our protein comes from animal sources, compared to just 7 percent in China. Most of their protein is plant protein. What we see is that by eating this type of diet, you can eat more food and more calories and still be leaner."

Banoo Parpia, Ph.D.
Senior Research Associate, China Health Project
Division of Nutritional Sciences
Cornell University
Ithica, New York

The Natural Approach

All of the natural remedies listed below can be used to supplement conventional medical treatment.

Herbal Medicine

Use one or more of the remedies listed below. For information on herbal medicine, see Chapter 2. Commercial preparations are also available; follow package directions.

• Coffee *(Coffea cruda):* While not usually considered an herbal remedy, coffee is actually a potent medicinal plant. Studies show that coffee boosts the number of calories you burn by about 4 percent per hour. Drinking coffee with a meal can increase the number of calories burned after the meal. To prepare an infusion (also known as brewing a cup of coffee), use 1 tablespoon of ground beans per cup of water, and brew using your favorite method. Drink up to three cups a day, unless you need to restrict caffeine intake in response to another medical condition.

- Dandelion *(Taraxacum officinale):* This herb has long been used to assist in weight loss by controlling water weight gain. Either eat fresh dandelion leaves in a salad, or prepare an infusion, using ½ ounce of dried leaves per cup of boiling water. Steep 10 minutes, strain, and drink up to three cups a day.

- Ephedra *(Ephedra sinica):* This herb is a powerful central nervous system stimulant, as well as a bronchial decongestant. It causes the body to burn calories faster, but it should not be used in combination with coffee, nasal decongestants, or any other stimulant. For a decoction, mix 1 teaspoon of dried herb per cup of water, bring to a boil, then simmer 10 to 15 minutes. Strain and drink up to two cups a day.

Diet and Nutrition Supplements

Note: Rather than focusing on overall calorie intake, try to follow a diet high in fiber, complex carbohydrates, fresh vegetables, and fruits; and low in fat and simple sugars. For information on nutrition supplements and good food sources of particular nutrients, see Chapter 3.

- Lecithin: This nutrition supplement helps break down fat in the body. Commercial products are available; follow package directions.

- Vitamin E: This vitamin is important for the metabolism of fat. Take 400 to 800 IU a day.

Homeopathy

Use one homeopathic treatment at a time, based on your specific symptoms. For information on homeopathy, see Chapter 4. For dosage information, see pages 56–57. Discontinue use if the symptoms disappear.

- Calcarea *(Calcarea carbonica)* 6c: Use if obesity is accompanied by indigestion, chills, and a sweaty head. One dose every 12 hours, for up to two weeks.
- Capsicum *(Capsicum annuum)* 6c: Use if obesity is accompanied by red face and burning stomach. One dose every 12 hours, for up to two weeks.
- Ferrum *(Ferrum metallicum)* 6c: Use if obesity is accompanied by paleness and oversensitivity. One dose every 12 hours, for up to two weeks.
- Graphites *(Graphites)* 6c: Use if obesity is accompanied by constipation, chills, skin problems, and eczema. One dose every 12 hours, for up to two weeks.
- Kali carb. *(Kali carbonicum)* 6c: Use if obesity is accompanied by backache and congestion. One dose every 12 hours, for up to two weeks.

Acupressure

Use one or more of the acupressure points listed below. For information on acupressure, see Chapter 5. For diagrams showing the specific pressure points, see pages 88–91.

- Conception Vessel 12: On the midline of the body, halfway between the base of the breastbone and the belly button. *Warning:* Don't use this point if you have a chronic or life-threatening illness, such as heart disease, cancer, or high blood pressure.
- Spleen 4: On the arch of the foot, one thumb-width from the ball of the foot, toward the heel.
- Spleen 16: On the lower edge of the rib cage, a half-inch in from the nipple line.

An Ounce of Prevention

You can avoid excessive weight gain by shedding extra pounds before things get out of hand. When the bathroom scale shows you weigh in at five pounds above your goal weight, it's time to watch your diet and exercise habits.

Also, be sure to drink at least eight 8-ounce glasses of water a day. The water helps keep the body hydrated, it helps with metabolism—and it's filling. (Try drinking a glass of water before you sit down to a meal if you feel you might be tempted to overindulge.)

Warning Signs

Though the extra pounds can sneak up on you, a weekly visit to the bathroom scale should provide ample warning. Another reminder of your changing physique may be the day-to-day fit of your clothing.

For More Information:

Nutrition for Optimal Health
P.O. Box 380
Winnetka, IL 60093
(708) 786-5326

Nutrition Education Association
P.O. Box 20301
3647 Glen Haven
Houston, TX 77225
(713) 665-2946

Osteoporosis

No matter what your age, now is the time to begin your battle against osteoporosis. Of course, it's best if you've consumed calcium-rich foods and exercised regularly your entire life to build strong bones, but it's never too late to start.

Osteoporosis, a medical condition that literally means "porous bones," affects about 25 million Americans—at least one out of every three women over age 60. (It is much less common and less severe in men, in part because their bones are one-third denser than women's to begin with.) The thin, brittle bones associated with osteoporosis can lead to broken hips, vertebrae, and other bones. In advanced cases a strong cough can break a rib, or a gentle bump can cause a fractured hip. In fact, nearly half a million older people take a fall each year that results in a broken hip caused at least in part by osteoporosis. These dangerous fractures leave many people unable to walk, and about 20 percent don't survive.

In most cases the problem arises when people have consumed too little calcium. The body needs this essential mineral for muscle contractions and other functions, so it "steals" from the bones, leaving them fragile and thin. Typically, people experience their peak bone mass in the spine at around age 30 and in the long bones at around age 35. After that, bone mass drops by about 1 percent a year, until a woman reaches menopause.

After menopause, bone loss speeds up to about 2 to 4 percent a year for the next ten years or so. (For every 10 percent loss in bone mass, your risk of bone fracture doubles.) Bone loss speeds up at menopause because the body has less estrogen, which helps the body absorb and use available calcium, and because the body produces less calcitonin, the hormone that prompts the bones to absorb calcium. (Estrogen replacement therapy can reduce the risk of osteoporosis fractures by up to 60 percent.) By the age of 80, most women have lost between a quarter and half their bone mass.

As the disease progresses, the spinal column may become compressed, causing the appearance of "shrinking." The spine may also curve, resulting in the characteristic "dowager's hump." These spinal changes actually result from fractures caused by the pressure of the body's weight on weak and brittle vertebrae.

In addition to dietary calcium deficiency, osteoporosis can also be caused by the inability to absorb enough calcium through the intestine, a calcium-phosphorus imbalance, a lack of exercise, and prolonged jaundice. Women at high risk include those with a thin frame, sedentary lifestyle, and a family history of the disease. Smokers, alcoholics, diabetics, women who reached menopause before age 40, those who consume a lot of caffeine, those who have never been pregnant, and Asian women and white women (especially blondes and redheads of Northern European ancestry) are also at increased risk. Certain drugs, such as cortisone, anticoagulants, anticonvulsants, and thyroid medications, can also contribute to calcium loss.

Conventional Care

Most doctors use X rays, blood tests, and bone-density tests to diagnose osteoporosis. (Unfortunately, the condition doesn't usually show up on X rays until there has been a 30 to 50 percent loss of bone.) A doctor may prescribe one of several drugs to prevent additional bone loss. Your doctor may also recommend estrogen replacement therapy; estrogen helps the bones absorb calcium. (For more information on estrogen replacement therapy, see pages 347–349.)

And of course, most doctors recommend lifestyle changes, including exercise and a calcium-rich diet. Studies have shown that it's never too late to exercise; one hour of moderate weight-bearing activity (such as walking) three times a week can actually increase bone mass, even in post-menopausal women. (For information on exercise, see Chapter 6.)

Words of Wisdom

"Every woman should know about wild yam, an herb. It is the precursor—the starting material—for natural progesterone, which helps prevent osteoporosis, PMS, and other menopausal symptoms."

Melinda Bonk
Member of the American Herbalists Guild
President, Wise Essentials
Minneapolis, Minnesota

The Natural Approach

All of the natural remedies listed below can be used to supplement conventional medical treatment. For more information on natural hormones, see the menopause section on page 340.

Herbal Medicine

Use one or more of the remedies listed below. For more information on herbal medicine, see Chapter 2. Commercial preparations are also available; follow package directions.

- Comfrey *(Symphytum officinale):* This herb, sometimes known as "knitbone," helps stimulate healing of tissues that have been damaged with a bone fracture. A comfrey compress can be made by mixing 3 tablespoons of powdered herb with 3 ounces of hot water. Apply the paste directly to the skin, and cover with a clean cloth for 2 or 3 hours. Commercially prepared salves and ointments are also available from health food stores.
- Horsetail *(Equisetum arvense):* This herb is good for bone repair. To make horsetail tea, simmer 2 teaspoons of the dried herb for 10 minutes in a cup of water. Steep for another 5 minutes, strain, and drink.
- Wild yam *(D. villosa):* This herb contains plant hormones similar to the hormone progesterone. In fact, until 1970 this plant was used in the manufacture of birth control pills. This herb is often used to treat menopausal symptoms, and it also helps preserve bone mass. It is commercially available from health food stores.

Diet and Nutrition Supplements

Use one or more of the remedies listed below. For information on nutrition supplements and good food sources of particular nutrients, see Chapter 3.

- Calcium: The primary cause of osteoporosis is calcium deficiency. Studies have shown that taking calcium supplements (with vitamin D) for only a year and a half dramatically decreases the number of bone fractures in women over age 80; women taking the supplements had 43 percent fewer hip fractures and 32 percent fewer fractures of the wrist, arm, and pelvis. Take 1,500 milligrams of calcium a day, either through dietary sources or supplements. (The average adult woman consumes one-third this amount.) You can boost the calcium content of many recipes without adding fat by adding powdered nonfat dry milk to recipes; every teaspoon of powdered milk adds about 50 milligrams of calcium.
- Magnesium: People with osteoporosis also tend to have low levels of magnesium. The ratio of calcium and magnesium should be balanced: too much calcium and too little magnesium can make the blood prone to clotting, contributing to stroke and heart attack. Take 750 milligrams of magnesium a day, aiming for about half as much magnesium as calcium.
- Soy: Soy-based foods contain phytoestrogens, or molecules very similar to estrogen and progesterone. In the body these estrogenlike substances help to protect the bones. Try to consume 25 grams of soy daily; a soy burger contains about 18 grams, a glass of soy milk about 8 grams. Powdered soy supplements are also available at health food stores.
- Vitamin D: The body needs vitamin D to absorb and use calcium. A good multivitamin should contain 400 IU of vitamin D, which is all you need.
- Zinc: The body needs zinc to utilize calcium and to support the immune system. Take up to 50 milligrams a day.

Foods to Avoid

To prevent osteoporosis, you need to consume more calcium—and to allow your body to use the calcium you do consume. Studies have shown that caffeine contributes to calcium loss and the leaching of important minerals from the bones. Limit your caffeine intake as much as possible; stick to just one cup of coffee a day, if you can. Likewise, high-protein diets can steal calcium from the body. Limit your protein intake to 6 ounces per day, roughly the amount of protein found in a small fish fillet or chicken breast.

Homeopathy

Use one homeopathic treatment at a time, based on your specific symptoms. For information on homeopathy, see Chapter 4. For dosage information, see pages 56–57. Discontinue use if the symptoms disappear.

- Arnica *(Arnica montana)* 30c: Use immediately after a bone fracture. One dose three times a day, for up to four days.
- Symphytum *(Symphytum officinale)* 6c: Use to promote healing of the bone. One dose twice a day, for up to three weeks.

Acupressure

Use one or more of the acupressure points listed below. For information on acupressure, see Chapter 5. For diagrams showing the specific pressure points, see pages 88–91.

- Bladder 10: A half-inch below the base of the skull on the band of muscles, a half-inch out from the spine.
- Bladder 48: Two finger-widths outside the large bony area at the base of the spine, midway between the top of the hipbone and the base of the buttock.
- Gallbladder 39: On the outside of the leg, four finger-widths above the tip of the anklebone, in the depression between the bone and the tendons.

An Ounce of Prevention

The best way to prevent osteoporosis is to build strong bones early in life and then take steps to keep bones healthy later in life. To minimize bone thinning, add calcium to your diet, either by eating more calcium-rich foods or by taking a supplement. The average American diet contains just 500 milligrams of calcium, but after menopause a woman needs about 1,500 milligrams.

In addition, build your bones through regular weight-bearing exercise, such as walking, bicycle riding, or dancing. Don't smoke or drink alcohol in excess, both of which can contribute to brittle bones. If you have had a bone fracture or are at high risk of developing osteoporosis, talk to your doctor about estrogen replacement, which can help to slow the development of the disease.

Warning Signs

Osteoporosis is a silent disease; it usually doesn't provide much advance warning. In fact, the first sign is often a severe hip or low-back pain, or a broken bone after a minor bump or fall. If you have sharp unexplained back pain that doesn't improve after two or three days, see your doctor.

Researchers have found that women with prematurely gray hair tend to develop osteoporosis more frequently than those who go gray later in life. While scientists do not fully understand why this is so, premature gray may offer an early warning of possible osteoporosis.

For More Information:

National Osteoporosis Foundation
1150 17th Street, N.W., Suite 500
Washington, DC 20036
(202) 223-2226
(800) 464-6700

National Women's Health Resource Center
2425 L Street, N.W.
Washington, DC 20037
(202) 293-6045

Osteoporosis Education Campaign
c/o The Older Women's League
666 11th Street, N.W., Suite 700
Washington, DC 20001
(202) 783-6686

What Type of Calcium?

Not all calcium is created equal. Different forms are absorbed by the body at different rates, so be sure to choose a type that your body can easily use.

For the body to use calcium, it must be ionized by stomach acid. Unfortunately, about 40 percent of postmenopausal women do not have enough stomach acid to do the job. Studies have found that women with low stomach acid absorb only about 4 percent of calcium taken as calcium carbonate (the most common form for supplements), compared with 22 percent for women with normal stomach acid.

Older women and those with low levels of stomach acid should take calcium citrate or calcium lactate, forms that arrive soluble, ionized, and ready for use. (It is also more bio-available to people with normal stomach acid.) Calcium citrate also lowers the risk of developing kidney stones, which can happen with other forms of calcium supplements.

Parkinson's Disease

Parkinson's is a paradoxical disease. When people suffer from it, some of their muscles become rigid and others contract involuntarily. People with Parkinson's disease may stoop, shuffle, and present a void, masklike, expressionless face, while at the same time suffer from an incessant tremor in the hand.

Parkinson's disease involves a failure of the body's internal communication system. When we are healthy, we take our bodies for granted, but every move we make, from kicking a ball to writing our names, requires thousands of coordinated communications between the brain, muscles, tendons, and bones. When these systems work well together, we think nothing of it, but when some part of the network breaks down, the effect can be devastating, as is the case with Parkinson's disease.

In 1817 British physician James Parkinson identified the disease that bears his name, though it was first called simply the "shaking palsy." The disease, which afflicts more than one million Americans, involves damage to the middle section of the brain known as the *substantia nigra*, named for its blackish pigmentation. This midbrain area is the main supplier of dopamine, the neurotransmitter that allows for communication about movement between various parts of the body. When these cells die off and the dopamine supply dwindles, the nerve signals cross and muscle action goes haywire.

Parkinson's is a degenerative disease that usually first show up when patients are in their fifties and sixties. There is no known cure for the disease, but the symptoms can be relieved through medication and natural treatments. Early treatment can help to slow the progress of the disease.

The cause of Parkinson's disease is unknown, though some experts suspect that either a virus, malnutrition, or chemical exposure could be involved. Supporting evidence for the virus-trigger theory is that many people who survived the encephalitis epidemics between 1919 and 1926 (caused by a virus) developed Parkinson's years later. The toxin-trigger theory was bolstered by evidence of an outbreak of a Parkinson's-like disorder among drug addicts in San Francisco in the early 1980s.

In some cases people develop symptoms of Parkinson's disease that prove actually to be side effects of medications. This is called Parkinson's syndrome rather than Parkinson's disease, and the symptoms disappear when the drugs are discontinued. If you suspect you have Parkinson's syndrome, review your use of all prescription and nonprescription drugs, and discuss the issue with your doctor.

Conventional Care

Since Parkinson's disease involves changes in brain chemistry, most treatments involve drug therapy, typically the use of the chemical L-dopa, which behaves in the body very much like dopamine, the missing neurotransmitter. Pay careful attention to warnings about food and drug interactions, which are common with drugs used to treat Parkinson's. In addition, some symptoms can be managed through physical and occupational therapy.

Words of Wisdom

"It's God and Nature against man and synthetics. That is really the battle. Evidence suggests that Parkinson's can be caused by exposure to toxins, so you can minimize your risk of developing Parkinson's—you can minimize your risk of all disease—by minimizing your exposure to toxins. We treat Parkinson's with nutrition and natural methods rather than heavy drugs. Establishment medicine will try synthetic drugs first and nutrition last. The closer to natural, the better."

James R. Priviera, M.D.
Covina, California

The Natural Approach

All of the natural remedies listed below can be used to supplement conventional medical treatment. Drug therapy should never be discontinued without the consent of your physician.

Diet and Nutrition Supplements

Use one or more of the remedies listed below. For information on nutrition supplements and good food sources of particular nutrients, see Chapter 3.

- Calcium and magnesium: These minerals are necessary for the transmission of nerve impulses; they should be taken in combination because they work together. Take up to 1,500 milligrams of calcium and 750 milligrams of magnesium a day.
- Vitamin C: This vitamin helps improve circulation in the brain; evidence also suggests that vitamin C's powerful antioxidant activity can protect the nerve cells

from damage. A recent study showed that 60 percent of elderly people with vitamin C deficiency had Parkinson's disease. Take up to 3,000 milligrams a day, in divided doses.

Homeopathy

Use one homeopathic treatment at a time, based on your specific symptoms. For information on homeopathy, see Chapter 4. For dosage information, see pages 56–57. Discontinue use if the symptoms disappear.

- Agaricus *(Agaricus muscarius)* 6c: Use when the limbs tremble or twitch and the person complains of stiffness. One dose every 6 hours, for up to two weeks.
- Hyoscyamus *(Hyoscyamus niger)* 6c: Use when person feels restless and twitchy. One dose every 6 hours, for up to two weeks.
- Mercurius *(Mercurius solubilis hahnemanni)* 6c: Use when there is drooling and an overproduction of saliva, as well as hand trembling. One dose every 6 hours, for up to two weeks.

An Ounce of Prevention

It's impossible to prevent Parkinson's because we do not understand its causes. Some experts suspect that environmental toxins and pesticides may play a role, but this link is not well established.

Warning Signs

Unfortunately, the early signs of Parkinson's include vague, minor symptoms that are often written off as typical signs of aging, including fatigue, stiffness, difficulty swallowing, and slight hand tremor. Classic Parkinson's symptoms—such as a constant "pill-rolling" motion of the fingers, a tendency to hold an arm with the elbow bent, small handwriting, and a "masklike" expression—tend to show up next. Finally, more severe signs appear, such as a slow, shuffling walk; severe tremor; stooped posture; muscle rigidity; and dementia.

For More Information:

Parkinson Support Groups of America
11376 Cherry Hill Road, No. 204
Beltsville, MD 20705
(301) 937-1545

Parkinson's Disease Foundation
William Black Medical Research Building
Columbia-Presbyterian Medical Center
650 West 168th Street
New York, NY 10032
(212) 923-4700

American Parkinson Disease Association
1250 Hylan Boulevard
Staten Island, NY 10305
(718) 981-8001
(800) 223-2732

United Parkinson Foundation
833 West Washington Boulevard
Chicago, Il 60607
(312) 733-1893

National Parkinson Foundation
1501 Northwest 9th Avenue
Miami, FL 33136
(800) 327-4545

Periodontal Disease

No matter what your age, a beautiful smile requires not only beautiful teeth but healthy gums. Periodontal disease (literally meaning "disease around the tooth") is the major cause of tooth loss in older people. To some degree, periodontal disease affects up to 85 percent of the population. The older you are, the more likely you are to have the problem; more than half of all Americans over age 50 have signs of gum disease.

The gums that surround your teeth are called gingiva, and the network of gums, bones, and ligaments that form the tooth socket are called the periodontium. When you develop periodontal disease, you can experience swollen, bleeding, and receding gums, as well as loose teeth.

Periodontal disease goes through three stages: gingivitis, periodontitis, and advanced periodontitis or pyorrhea. Stage 1 (gingivitis) refers to inflammation of the gums caused by plaque, the sticky bacterial film that forms on the teeth and gums. Plaque continuously builds up on the teeth, where it causes no harm as long as it is removed within twenty-four hours or so. After that time the plaque hardens into tartar (also known as calculus), which in turn produces toxins and enzymes that irritate the gums, causing them to become red and swollen. The gums may also bleed during brushing and flossing and begin to recede from the tooth.

If treated at this stage, periodontal disease can be controlled, since it has not yet damaged the bone and ligaments that hold the teeth in place. Untreated, however, the disease progresses to stage 2 (periodontitis) in which the plaque slips beneath the gums and begins to damage the roots of the teeth. Again, without proper treatment, the disease advances to stage 3 (advanced periodontitis or pyorrhea), which affects the bones and support system for the teeth. In stage 3, the gums often recede to the point that the teeth appear elongated; pockets form underneath the gums, where additional plaque and food can collect, causing bad breath and greater gum irritation. The plaque and tartar under the gum line can cause infections that damage the bone, resulting in loose teeth and the loss of teeth.

While inadequate tooth cleaning is the major cause of periodontal disease, other contributing factors include habitual clenching and grinding of the teeth, mouth breathing, a high-sugar diet, and the use of tobacco, drugs, and alcohol. Heredity, hormonal imbalances, and stress are other possible factors.

Conventional Care

The best way to manage gum disease is to keep the teeth and gums in tip-top shape by brushing and flossing them regularly and getting regular professional cleanings. Each stage of gum disease needs a different type of professional cleaning. (Cleanings and checkups may be required four times a year in many cases.)

During a periodontal visit the doctor uses a periodontal probe to assess the degree of gum damage, then cleans the surface of the teeth. In more advanced cases, where plaque and tartar have built up under the gums and on the root of the tooth, a scaler must be used to scrape away the debris under the gum line.

Words of Wisdom

"Gum erosion is common, but it isn't necessarily inevitable. I have patients who are in their seventies and eighties who have beautiful teeth and gums. The two most important factors are things that people have heard before: They need to clean between their teeth every day—mainly by flossing—and they need to see their dentist regularly. If those two simple things were done, people would have a lot less gum disease and tooth decay."

David L. Stephenson, D.D.S., L.Ac.
Anaheim, California

The Natural Approach

All of the natural remedies listed below can be used to supplement conventional medical treatment.

Herbal Medicine

Use one or more of the remedies listed below. For information on herbal medicine, see Chapter 2. Commercial preparations are also available; follow package directions.

- Aloe vera *(Aloe vera):* Gel of the aloe vera plant helps soothe throbbing gums and heal inflamed tissue. Apply the gel directly to the gums before bed.
- Goldenseal *(Hydrastis canadensis):* This herb helps reverse gums disease. Mix one teaspoon of goldenseal powder with enough water to form a thick paste, then gently brush your teeth and gums.

Diet and Nutrition Supplements

Use one or more of the remedies listed below. Some vitamins can be used topically, as noted. For information on nutrition supplements and good food sources of particular nutrients, see Chapter 3.

- Calcium: Strong, healthy bones and teeth need plenty of calcium. Take up to 1,500 milligrams a day.
- Magnesium: Calcium and magnesium work together to promote healthy teeth and gums. Take 750 milligrams a day.
- Vitamin C: This vitamin is critical to the formation of connective tissue; it also promotes healing of bleeding, unhealthy gums. Take 1,500 to 3,000 milligrams a day in divided doses.
- Vitamin E: When gums are inflamed, open a capsule of vitamin E oil and rub it directly on the affected area to relieve soreness and promote healing.
- Zinc: Periodontal disease has been linked to zinc deficiency. Zinc also promotes wound healing. Take up to 50 milligrams a day.

Homeopathy

Use one homeopathic treatment at a time, based on your specific symptoms. For information on homeopathy, see Chapter 4. For dosage information, see pages 56–57. Discontinue use if the symptoms disappear.

- Kali phos. *(Kali phosphoricum)* 6x: Use when the gums are spongy and receding and bleed easily. One dose three times daily.
- Kreosotum *(Creosote)* 6c: Use when the gums are swollen, red, and bleed easily, with the roots of the teeth exposed. One dose every 4 hours, for up to three days.
- Mercurius corr. *(Mercurius corrosivus)* 6x: Use when the gums are swollen and the teeth feel loose. One dose three times daily.
- Phosphorus *(Phosphorus)* 6c: Use when the gums

bleed easily when touched. One dose every 4 hours, for up to three days.

Acupressure

Use one or more of the acupressure points listed below. For information on acupressure, see Chapter 5. For diagrams showing the specific pressure points, see pages 88–91.

- Gallbladder 2: Just behind the jawbone and in front of the earlobe, in the depression formed when the mouth is open.
- Governing Vessel 26: In the center of the tissue between the upper lip and the bottom on the nose. *Note:* Do not use this point if you have high blood pressure.
- Stomach 3: Just below the cheekbone, directly below the pupil of the eye and level with the outside edge of the nostril.
- Stomach 6: Along the lower angle of the jawbone, in the depression formed by the muscles and tendons when the teeth are clenched.

An Ounce of Prevention

You've heard it before, you'll hear it again: To prevent gum disease and tooth decay, brush and floss your teeth daily. Gum disease usually stems from plaque buildup, so be diligent about brushing your teeth after every meal, if possible. (If you can't brush, at least rinse well with water.) Some dentists believe an electric toothbrush stimulates the gums, in addition to cleaning the teeth, so consider using one if your dentist recommends it. Avoid mouthwashes with alcohol, which can dry out and irritate sensitive gums. And of course, have your teeth professionally cleaned twice a year, or more often if you already have periodontal disease.

Warning Signs

You may develop periodontal disease without knowing it.
Discuss the health of your gums when you visit your dentist
for regular checkups. Between dental appointments, look
for signs of swollen or bleeding gums, which can also indicate gum problems.

For More Information:

American Academy of Periodontology
737 North Michigan Avenue, Suite 800
Chicago, IL 60611-2615
(312) 787-5518

American Board of Periodontology
Baltimore College of Dental Surgery
University of Maryland
666 West Baltimore Street
Baltimore, MD 21201
(410) 706-2432

American Dental Association
211 East Chicago Avenue
Chicago, IL 60611
(312) 440-2500

Pneumonia

Many older people live in fear that every cough or cold may slip into pneumonia. In fact, this fear is not misplaced. The prospect of a cold or flu becoming a serious infection is a very real health threat for older people, especially those whose resistance is down. In fact, pneumonia is the fifth leading cause of death among people over age 65.

A number of different bacteria, viruses, and fungi can trigger pneumonia. Pneumonia is actually an infection of the alveoli, the tiny air sacs in the lungs, which become inflamed and then fill with mucus and pus. When infected, the alveoli cannot do their job of transferring oxygen from the lungs to the blood, so the person feels tired and out of breath. Other symptoms of pneumonia include fever, chills, cough, sweating, chest pain, rapid breathing, and enlarged lymph glands in the neck. If the body is denied enough oxygen, the lips, fingernails, and toenails may turn somewhat blue.

Pneumonia often follows a cold, flu, bronchitis, or another upper respiratory tract infection. It can also be caused by stroke, alcoholism, smoking, kidney failure, sickle-cell disease, malnutrition, foreign bodies in the respiratory passages, chemical irritation, and allergies. Pneumonia is a serious illness that should be treated by a physician, though you can also use natural remedies to help manage your symptoms.

Conventional Care

To diagnose pneumonia, your doctor will listen to your chest as you breathe, checking for evidence of crackling noises, which indicate the disease. Chest X rays can then confirm the diagnosis. Laboratory tests of sputum samples may be analyzed to confirm the type of infection. For bacterial infections, your doctor will prescribe antibiotics (such as penicillin or erythromycin); for viral infections, he or she may prescribe other drugs.

In addition, you will be asked to drink plenty of fluids to loosen the phlegm, and you may use massage, heat treatments, and expectorants to release the secretions so that they can be coughed up. In severe cases your doctor may recommend hospitalization, so that oxygen and artificial ventilation are available, if necessary. Six weeks after recovery, a follow-up chest X ray should be done to ensure that the infection has cleared.

The Natural Approach

All of the natural remedies listed below can be used to supplement conventional medical treatment.

Herbal Medicine
Use one or more of the remedies listed below. For information on herbal medicine, see Chapter 2. Commercial preparations are also available; follow package directions.

- Herbal expectorant: This combination of several herbs works as a natural expectorant, thinning the secretions in the lungs and allowing them to be more readily coughed up and removed. To prepare an herbal expectorant, combine 2 ounces of licorice root *(Glycyrrhiza glabra)*, 1 ounce of wild cherry bark *(Prunus serotina)*, and 1 ounce of horehound *(Marrubium vultgare)*. Add 4 cups of water, and boil for 2 minutes, then let it steep for 10 minutes. Strain and take one cup every 2 hours. (Sweeten with honey if necessary.)
- Hyssop *(Hyssopus officinalis):* This herb has long been used to "cleanse the lungs" and to treat chest congestion. It contains a chemical that acts as expectorant. For an infusion, use 2 teaspoons of dried herb per cup of boiling water. Steep 10 minutes; strain and drink, up to three cups a day. Commercially prepared products are available; follow package directions.

Diet and Nutrition Supplements

Use one or more of the remedies listed below. For information on nutrition supplements and good food sources of particular nutrients, see Chapter 3.

- Fluids: Drink at least the recommended eight 8-ounce glasses of water a day—or more if you can stand it. Fluids help to thin the secretions in the lungs, making coughing more productive.
- Vitamin A: This vitamin helps maintain the health of the lining of the respiratory passages. Vitamin A deficiency increases the susceptibility to respiratory infections and pneumonia. Take a multivitamin, which should include an adequate supply of vitamin A.
- Vitamin C: This vitamin reduces inflammation, boosts the immune response, and helps ward off pneumonia, especially if taken on the first or second day of infection. Take 1,000 to 3,000 milligrams a day, in divided doses.
- Zinc: Proper immune function and tissue repair de-

pends on adequate levels of zinc in the body. Suck on zinc lozenges, following package directions for dosage information.

Homeopathy

Use one homeopathic treatment at a time, based on your specific symptoms. For information on homeopathy, see Chapter 4. For dosage information, see pages 56–57. Discontinue use if the symptoms disappear.

- Bryonia *(Bryonia alba)* 30c: Use if pneumonia is accompanied by sharp chest pains. One dose every 2 hours, for up to ten doses.
- Phosphorus *(Phosphorus)* 6c: Use if the cough is accompanied by brown- or rust-colored sputum. One dose every 2 hours, for up to ten doses.
- Sanguinaria *(Sanguinaria canadensis)* 6c: Use if pneumonia follows the flu, or if the phlegm is bloody and difficult to bring up. One dose every 2 hours, for up to ten doses.

Acupressure

For information on acupressure, see page Chapter 5. For diagrams showing the specific pressure point, see pages 88–91.

- Lung 9: On the inside of the wrist, along the wrist crease and in the depression beneath the bone at the base of the thumb.

An Ounce of Prevention

If you haven't had a vaccine against pneumonia and you're in good health and over age 65, call your doctor to schedule an appointment to be immunized. (Also talk to your doctor about the vaccine if you're under 65 but have an increased risk of developing pneumonia because you have

Hodgkin's disease, an immune disorder, or heart, kidney, liver or lung disease.)

A single injection of the vaccine provides lifelong immunity against about 90 percent of the types of bacteria that cause pneumococcal infections in the United States. It also helps protect against bacteremia (infections of the bloodstream) and meningitis (infections of the covering of the brain and spinal column). Despite its obvious benefits and widespread availability, only one out of every four Americans over 65 has received this life-saving vaccine. As a result, more than 268,000 older people develop pneumococcal disease and nearly 33,000 die from it every year, even though these deaths could be prevented.

Side effects of the vaccine include pain and mild swelling at the injection site in about half the people who receive it. Fever, muscle pain, and more serious local reactions occur in fewer than one percent of people receiving the shot. You can get the pneumococcal vaccine at the same time as a flu shot with no adverse effects.

In addition to getting the vaccine, you may be able to avoid pneumonia in some cases by building and maintaining your body's resistance to disease by eating a balanced diet and getting plenty of rest and exercise. Also be sure to take care of colds and flu (for information, see page 213), so that these relatively minor illnesses do not develop into pneumonia.

Warning Signs

In the early stages it's difficult to tell the difference between a bad cold and pneumonia. But if a cough following a cold lingers for more than a week, if your fever reaches 101 degrees F or higher, if you cough up green, yellow, or brown sputum, or if you experience rapid or labored breathing, call your doctor. These warning signs indicate that you're dealing with more than a common cold.

Ulcers

At first you may have thought it was a bad case of heartburn or indigestion. But when the burning pain failed to subside, you suspected much worse: an ulcer.

At least five million Americans suffer from ulcers, or open sores or lesions in the lining of the gastrointestinal tract. Ulcers form when there is too much stomach acid or when the mucous lining fails to protect the digestive tract. Older adults who take large doses of stomach-irritating, anti-inflammatory drugs to manage their arthritis pain are at increased risk for ulcers.

There are two kinds of ulcers: gastric, which appear in the stomach, and duodenal, which form in the duodenum (the first part of the small intestine). It is possible to have both kinds of ulcers at the same time. Ulcers often form during times of stress, when the stomach cannot secrete enough mucus to protect itself from the strong acids used for digestion.

New research also suggests that many ulcers are caused or exacerbated by a bacterium known as *Helicobacter pylori*. A two-week regimen of antibiotics can wipe out this bacterium, vastly diminishing the odds of a recurrence. More than 70 percent of ulcer sufferers are believed to be infected with the bacterium. In one study 95 percent of the people who took antibiotics as part of their treatment remained ulcer-free for two years, compared with only 12 percent of those who had standard treatment without antibiotics.

Left untreated or undetected, ulcers can lead to peritonitis, an inflammation of the lining of the abdominal cavity. In severe cases an ulcer can burn a hole right through the stomach or intestine; this is a medical emergency. Fortunately, a number of natural remedies can be used to prevent and treat ulcers before they reach this stage.

Conventional Care

You need to visit your doctor to confirm the diagnosis of an ulcer. To determine the presence, location, and severity of the ulcer, your doctor may use an X ray or view the lesion directly through a gastroscope, in which a tube is threaded through the mouth into the intestinal tract. Additional tests may be performed to analyze stomach acid and to test for internal bleeding.

Treatment typically includes antibiotics to kill ulcer-causing bacteria and antacids and other drugs to neutralize gastric acids. (Most antacids contain a lot of sodium; they should be used with caution by people on low-sodium diets and by people with high blood pressure. Some antacids also contain glucose, which should be noted by diabetics and others who need to watch their sugar intake.) If the ulcer doesn't heal within eight weeks, surgery may be recommended to remove the ulcerated portion of the stomach.

The Natural Approach

All of the natural remedies listed below can be used to supplement conventional medical treatment.

Herbal Medicine

Use one or more of the remedies listed below. For information on herbal medicine, see Chapter 2. Commercial preparations are also available; follow package directions.

- Chamomile *(Matricaria chamomilla):* This herb helps prevent and heal ulcers. For an infusion, use 2 to 3 heaping teaspoons of flowers per cup of boiling water; steep 10 to 20 minutes. Strain, and drink up to three cups a day. Commercial preparations are also available; follow package directions.
- Licorice *(Glycyrrhiza glabra):* DGL (deglycyrrhizinated licorice), an extract of the licorice herb, heals ulcers without causing the serious side effects associated with the herb, especially high blood pressure. A three-month study of duodenal-ulcer sufferers found that DGL healed ulcers faster than the popular drug Tagamet. Commercially prepared DGL products are available; follow package directions.

Diet and Nutrition Supplements

Use one or more of the remedies listed below. For information on nutrition supplements and good food sources of particular nutrients, see Chapter 3.

- Cabbage juice: Raw cabbage juice can be remarkably successful in treating ulcers. One liter per day of the fresh juice, taken in divided doses, results in total ulcer healing in an average of just ten days. The high glutamine content of the juice is probably responsible for its efficacy.
- High-fiber diet: A high-fiber diet is associated with a reduced rate of duodenal ulcer; it also cuts recurrence

rate of the illness. Fiber promotes the secretion of mucus, which helps protect the digestive tract.

- Zinc: Zinc increases mucin production and has been shown to have a protective effect against peptic ulcers in animals and a protective effect in humans. Take up to 50 milligrams a day.

Foods to Avoid

Contrary to popular belief, you should pass on the milk if you have an ulcer. Even though milk helps neutralize stomach acid, the calcium and protein in it stimulate the production of more acid, creating a "rebound" effect.

Acupressure

Use one or more of the acupressure points listed below. For information on acupressure, see Chapter 5. For diagrams showing the specific pressure points, see pages 88–91.

- Conception Vessel 12: On the midline of the body, three finger-widths below the base of the breastbone, in the pit of the upper stomach.
- Spleen 16: On the lower edge of the rib cage, at the junction of the ninth rib cartilage to the eighth rib, a half-inch in from the nipple line.

An Ounce of Prevention

To minimize the risk of ulcers, eat six small meals a day rather than three larger ones. The presence of food can help to neutralize stomach acid, so don't go too long without eating. Eliminate alcohol, and minimize your intake of caffeine. Also take steps to manage stress, which can increase the production of stomach acid. Quit smoking; tobacco smoke constricts the blood vessels lining the stomach, making the stomach wall more vulnerable to sores.

Warning Signs

Symptoms of a duodenal or peptic ulcer include a burning pain just above the navel (especially when the stomach is empty), heartburn, and nausea. The pain may wake you up in the middle of the night. Often eating a slice of plain bread will ease the pain by absorbing the acid, but the pain often reappears an hour or so later when the body produces more acid. Yet only about 50 percent of all people with stomach ulcers have telltale symptoms.

Seek immediate medical care if you vomit blood or material that looks like coffee grounds. Also seek help if black, tarry blood appears in the stool. These are signs that the ulcer is bleeding, which can cause anemia. Blood can also indicate a perforated ulcer, one that has burned through the stomach or intestinal wall.

For More Information:

National Digestive Disease Information Clearinghouse
2 Information Way
Bethesda, MD 20892-3570
(301) 654-3810

Digestive Disease National Coalition
711 2nd Street, N.E., Suite 200
Washington, DC 20002
(202) 544-7497

Center for Ulcer Research and Education Foundation
11301 Wilshire Boulevard
Los Angeles, CA 90073
(310) 312-9283

Vaginal Dryness

It's not your fault—or your partner's—if you lack vaginal lubrication during sex after menopause. Vaginal dryness is a normal physiological change associated with growing older and passing through menopause, but it need not interfere with your sexual appetite or pleasure.

Sexual arousal increases the blood flow to the vagina, releasing secretions that lubricate it in preparation for sexual intercourse. After menopause estrogen levels drop, and the walls of the vagina tend to become thinner and drier. (Vaginal dryness can also be caused by taking birth control pills, or by the presence of a vaginal infection.) Vaginal dryness can make sexual intercourse less comfortable—or in some cases downright painful and irritating—but fortunately, steps can be taken to restore vaginal moisture and lubrication.

Conventional Care

All it takes to restore vaginal moisture in most cases is a quick trip to the drugstore to buy lubricating jelly. Look for a product that is water soluble, unscented, and colorless. (Vegetable oil also works, if you eschew commercial products.) Avoid petroleum-based products, such as Vaseline, which can cause irritation and damage condoms. (Some women continue to have their partners use condoms to prevent the spread of sexually transmitted diseases even after the threat of pregnancy has passed.) Some medical doctors may prescribe a vaginal estrogen cream to restore the condition of the vaginal tissues.

In addition, regular sexual activity (two or three sexual encounters a week) can improve blood circulation to the vagina and help to restore moisture. Hormone replacement therapy also relieves symptoms. (See pages 347–349 for a complete discussion of hormone replacement therapy.)

Words of Wisdom

"The baby boomers are turning 50 and 51 and going through menopause, and a lot of them are looking for alternatives to conventional medicine. Natural hormones, such as those found in wild yam, are the answer. They can take care of the vaginal dryness—as well as most other problems of menopause—and they're much safer than synthetic hormones. Women should know that they do have choices. There's no reason for women to experience vaginal dryness at any age."

Marjorie Moore-Jones, M.Ed., L.Ac., Dip. AAPM
Tustin, California

The Natural Approach

All of the natural remedies listed below can be used to supplement conventional medical treatment. For more information on natural hormones, see the menopause section on page 340.

Herbal Medicine

For information on herbal medicine, see Chapter 2.

- Wild yam *(D. villosa):* This herb contains plant hormones very similar to the female hormone progesterone. In fact, until 1970, this plant was used in the manufacture of birth control pills. This herb is often used to treat menopausal symptoms, including vaginal dryness. Powdered herb (for internal use) is available from health food stores.

Diet and Nutrition Supplements

For information on nutrition supplements and good food sources of particular nutrients, see Chapter 3.

- Soy: Soybeans and soy products contain phytoestrogens, or molecules very similar to estrogen and progesterone. A menopausal woman who eats a diet rich in soy protein can retain vaginal moisture and other benefits she had previously received from her body's natural estrogen. Try to consume 25 grams of soy daily; a soy burger contains about 18 grams, a glass of soy milk about 8 grams. Powdered soy supplements are also available at health food stores.
- Vitamin E: Vitamin E can help prevent vaginal dryness. Take 400 to 800 IU daily.

Homeopathy

For information on homeopathy, see Chapter 4. For dosage information, see pages 56–57. Discontinue use if the symptoms disappear.

- Bryonia *(Bryonia alba)* 30c: Use when vaginal dryness is accompanied by constipation. One dose twice a day, for up to one week.

Acupressure

Use one or more of the acupressure points listed below. For information on acupressure, see Chapter 5. For diagrams showing the specific pressure points, see pages 88–91.

- Conception Vessel 6: Two finger-widths below the navel, in the center of the abdomen.
- Gallbladder 26: On the side of the abdomen, below the eleventh rib.
- Governing Vessel 4: On the spine, between the second and third lumbar vertebrae.

An Ounce of Prevention

In many cases vaginal dryness can be overcome by allowing plenty of time for foreplay and sexual arousal before intercourse. (Keep in mind that sexual response tends to occur more slowly after menopause.) Vaginal lubrication also can be increased by boosting blood circulation to the vagina through the regular practice of Kegel exercises, which also promotes vaginal muscle tone and helps prevent urinary incontinence. (For information on Kegel exercises, see page 331.)

Warning Signs

Vaginal dryness is usually a harmless—though sometimes an uncomfortable and embarrassing—problem. But if the dryness results in vaginal bleeding during intercourse or is accompanied by severe itching, consult a health professional to rule out other problems.

For More Information:

Society for Menstrual Cycle Research
10559 North 104th Plaza
Scottsdale, AZ 85258
(602) 451-9731

North American Menopause Society
c/o University Hospitals of Cleveland
Dept. OB/GYN
Room 7024
1110 Euclid Avenue
Cleveland, OH 44106
(216) 844-8748

Varicose Veins

Varicose veins are nothing to be ashamed of, even though many people go to great lengths to hide them. In fact, more than 40 million Americans live with the swollen and sometimes painful veins, which most often appear in the legs.

Gravity is to blame for the formation of varicose veins. Blood that circulates to the legs must be pumped uphill to the heart, against the pull of gravity. Veins are equipped with one-way valves to prevent the blood from flowing back down the legs, but when the valves are stretched or damaged, they don't close properly, and the blood slips back down and pools, causing the veins to stretch out and appear blue and puffy.

Women experience varicose veins about four times more often than men, partially because of the rigors of pregnancy and childbirth. In preparation for childbirth a pregnant woman's body releases hormones that weaken the collagen and connective tissues in the pelvis to make the birth process easier. But these hormones can also weaken the collagen and valves in the veins, increasing the likelihood of varicose veins. Other common causes of varicose veins include standing for long periods (the pressure exerted against the veins can increase up to ten times when standing), and sitting for long periods without movement, especially with the legs crossed. (The leg muscles aren't being used to help push the blood back up toward the heart.) Genetics and obesity also contribute to the problem.

While some people consider varicose veins unsightly, they do not pose a health risk in most cases, when the affected veins are near the skin surface. Varicose veins that form deep within the leg, however, can lead to more serious complications, such as skin ulcers, phlebitis (inflammation of the vein), and thrombosis (formation of a blood clot). These conditions require immediate medical attention.

Conventional Care

In many cases doctors recommend that people with varicose veins wear elastic compression stockings, which squeeze the legs and prevent the pooling of blood in the veins. These surgical stockings are available at most pharmacies, but stockings from surgical supply houses are often more effective.

In severe cases a doctor may suggest using one of several techniques to destroy the affected vein. (The surrounding veins rapidly take the place of the one that has been eliminated, so there is no damage to the surrounding tissue.) One method involves injecting the vein with sclerosing agents, which close off the vein. The affected vein can also be surgically removed though a process known as vein stripping, in which the vein is removed through a small incision.

Keep in mind that even after veins have been destroyed

or removed, the relief may only be temporary. The best way to control the situation is to prevent the formation of new varicose veins through the use of exercise, diet, and natural remedies.

The Natural Approach

All of the natural remedies listed below can be used to supplement conventional medical treatment.

Herbal Medicine

Use one or more of the remedies listed below. For more information on herbal medicine, see Chapter 2. Commercial preparations are also available; follow package directions.

- Butcher's broom *(Ruscus aculeatus):* This herb contains ruscogenins, compounds known to fight inflammation and constrict the veins. Follow package directions when taking commercially prepared tinctures.
- Gotu kola *(Centella asiatica):* Clinical studies have shown that gotu kola extract helps improve varicose veins, probably because it enhances connective tissue structure and improves blood flow. For an infusion, use ½ teaspoon of dried herb per cup of boiling water. Strain, and drink up to two cups a day. Commercially prepared tinctures are also available; follow package directions.
- Horse chestnut *(Aesculus hippocastanum):* This herb fights inflammation, decreases the number and size of the small pores of the capillary walls, and tones the walls of the veins by strengthening their elastic fibers. Commercially prepared tinctures are available; follow package directions. The tincture can also be diluted with one part water and used in a topical compress for 10 to 15 minutes three or four times a day.
- King's clover *(Melilotus officinalis):* This herb is a

good venous tonic, an anticoagulant and anti-inflammatory. Commercially prepared tinctures are available; follow package directions.
- Witch hazel *(Hamamelis virginiana):* This astringent
herb can be soothing when applied topically. Commercially prepared tinctures are available; follow
package directions.

Diet and Nutrition Supplements

Use one or more of the remedies listed below. For information on nutrition supplements and good food sources of
particular nutrients, see Chapter 3.

- Flavonoids: Flavonoid-rich berries, such as hawthorn
berries, cherries, blueberries, and blackberries, help
prevent and treat varicose veins by strengthening the
walls of the veins. Eat two or three servings of these
richly colored berries a day.
- High-fiber diet: Varicose veins may be exacerbated
by a low-fiber diet, which can result in straining during bowel movements. Over time the straining
may weaken the vein walls, resulting in varicose veins
or hemorrhoids (which are varicose veins in the
anus). Eat a high-fiber diet rich in vegetables, fruits,
legumes, and grains.
- Vitamin C: This vitamin aids circulation by reducing
the tendency for blood clots to form. Take up to 3,000
milligrams a day, in divided doses.
- Vitamin E: This vitamin improves circulation and
helps prevent a heavy feeling in the legs. Take 400 to
800 IU a day.

Homeopathy

Use one homeopathic treatment at a time, based on your
specific symptoms. For information on homeopathy, see
Chapter 4. For dosage information, see pages 56–57. Discontinue use if the symptoms disappear.

- Hamamelis *(Hamamelis virginiana)* 30c: Use when the affected veins feel sore and swollen, with a burning sensation. The condition feels worse in warm, humid weather and with movement. One dose twice a day, for up to seven days.
- Pulsatilla *(Pulsatilla nigricans)* 30c: Use when varicose veins first appear during pregnancy and the veins feel worse when the legs hang down. One dose twice daily, for up to seven days.

Acupressure

Use one or more of the acupressure points listed below. For information on acupressure, see Chapter 5. For diagrams showing the specific pressure points, see pages 88–91.

- Kidney 6: One thumb-width below the inside of the anklebone.
- Spleen 6: On the inside of the leg, four finger-widths above the tip of the anklebone and just inside the bone of the leg.
- Spleen 9: On the inside of the leg, below the knee and under the large bulge of bone.
- Spleen 10: On the inside edge of the top of the knee, where the opposite thumb touches the muscles when the knee is flexed.

An Ounce of Prevention

You can reduce your risk of developing varicose veins by avoiding: standing for long periods of time, crossing your legs, lifting heavy objects, and wearing tight shoes, garters, or undergarments. Regular exercise—especially walking, biking, and jogging—helps to prevent varicose veins and to combat them once they have formed; the contraction of the leg muscles helps move the pooled blood in the legs back into circulation.

Warning Signs

Before varicose veins appear, some people experience a slight tingling on the surface of the leg caused by the reduced blood flow as the vein weakens. Others don't notice any change until they look down one day and spot a ropy blue vein bulging from their legs near the surface of the skin. Other symptoms include a heavy feeling in the legs, swollen ankles, leg cramps at night, and itchy, scaly skin near the affected areas.

If you experience sharp leg pains or notice a red lump in the vein that doesn't go away when you put your legs up, contact your doctor immediately. You may have a blood clot, which can lead to serious medical problems, including stroke.

Wrinkles

You can't win the war against wrinkles, but you can put up a good fight. Wrinkles are a natural part of the aging process. After about age 25, the cells in the dermis—the deeper layers of the skin—begin to shrink and die off. Over the years, the skin loses elasticity and becomes stiffer, making it prone to wrinkles when it is stretched. Frowning and chronic squinting can contribute to wrinkling, but the biggest culprits are smoking, sun exposure, alcohol consumption, and poor diet.

Conventional Care

Over-the-counter cosmetics and moisturizers promise beauty in a jar. Many wrinkle-fighting products contain Retin-A, a medication used to treat acne that has become a popular topical treatment for wrinkles. If you choose to use products containing Retin-A, heed the warnings carefully; Retin-A can cause skin rash and sun sensitivity.

Other popular wrinkle creams are those containing alpha-hydroxy acids (such as glycolic acid, lactic acid, or malic acid). These acids occur naturally in sour milk, citrus fruits, and sugar cane. These creams tend to have fewer side effects than Retin-A. Both Retin-A and products containing alpha-hydroxy acids can be effective in reducing tiny wrinkles, but they cannot reverse the aging process.

If over-the-counter products aren't effective enough, you can seek professional help. Medical treatment for wrinkles involves chemical face peels, dermabrasion, collagen injections, microlipoinjections (fat injections or transfers), and face-lifts.

The Natural Approach

All of the natural remedies listed below can be used to supplement conventional medical treatment.

Herbal Medicine

For information on herbal medicine, see Chapter 2. Commercial preparations are also available.

- Aloe vera *(Aloe vera):* The gel from this plant helps heal cell damage to the skin. It can be used directly from the leaves of the plant.
- Peppermint: A tea made with peppermint leaves and apple cider vinegar can be used as a facial rinse for dry skin. Add 1 teaspoon of dried peppermint leaves to 1 cup of hot water; steep for 10 minutes. Add 1 cup of apple cider vinegar. Cool and use as a rinse after washing; apply a final rinse of cool water.

Diet and Nutrition Supplements

For information on nutrition supplements and good food sources of particular nutrients, see Chapter 3.

- Vitamin A: This antioxidant helps minimize cell damage and maintain healthy skin. Take up to 10,000 IU of vitamin A daily.
- Vitamin B complex: The B vitamins are essential for healthy skin. In fact, cracks around the lips can be a sign of B-vitamin deficiency. Eat foods high in B vitamins, such as chicken, eggs, and whole wheat, and take a multivitamin with a B complex.
- Vitamin C: This vitamin helps the skin remain supple by repairing connective tissue. Take up to 1,500 milligrams a day in divided doses.
- Vitamin E: This antioxidant aids in skin repair. Take 400 to 800 IU daily. Vitamin E can also be applied directly to the skin.
- Water: Drink at least eight 8-ounce glasses of water each day to prevent dehydration and dry skin.

An Ounce of Prevention

It is much easier to prevent skin damage than to try to reverse it. The following tips can help:

- Stay out of the sun. Tanning really is the enemy of the skin. Avoid direct sunlight at midday—from 10 A.M. to 2 P.M.—and stay out of the tanning booth.
- Always use a sunscreen with a 15 or higher SPF—Sun Protection Factor. Protect your skin every day, not just when you're headed for the beach.
- Don't smoke. Though there are many other good reasons to quit smoking, if vanity is what it takes to help you kick the habit, so be it. Smoking causes premature wrinking; if you smoke a pack and a half of cigarettes a day, your skin will look about ten years older than the skin of a nonsmoker, other factors being equal. (The nicotine in the cigarette smoke constricts the blood vessels, interfering with the flow of oxygen and nutrients to the cells in the skin. The act of smoking

also causes you to purse your lips when you draw in the smoke, causing additional facial wrinkles.)

- Wear moisturizer. No, moisturizer cannot reverse wrinkling, but it can make the skin temporarily appear smoother.
- Wash with mild soaps and cleansers that won't dry out your skin or strip away all the natural oils.
- Pass on the booze. Drinking alcohol causes facial swelling, which stretches the skin and contributes to wrinkling. The alcohol also depletes the body of nutrients that promote healthy skin.
- Reach your optimal weight—and stay there. Weight gain and loss can contribute to saggy skin.
- Work out those wrinkles. Exercise increases circulation to the skin and improves oxygen supply to the tissues.

Warning Signs

Wrinkles can sometimes be a harbinger of future skin problems. If you have premature wrinkling as a result of sun exposure, you should be on the lookout for signs of skin cancer, which can be caused by exposure to the sun's rays.

Appendix A: Additional Reading

Balch, James F., M.D. and Phyllis A. Balch, C.N.C. *Prescription for Nutritional Healing.* Garden City Park, N.Y.: Avery Publishing Group, 1990.

Bauer, Cathryn. *Acupressure for Everybody.* New York: Henry Holt and Company, 1991.

Bauer, Cathryn. *Acupressure for Women.* Freedom, Calif.: The Crossing Press, 1987.

Beers, Mark H., M.D., and Stephen K. Urice, Ph.D., J.D. *Aging in Good Health: A Complete, Essential Medical Guide for Older Men and Women and Their Families.* New York: Pocket Books, 1992.

Bricklin, Mark, *The Practical Encyclopedia of Natural Healing.* Emmaus, Pa.: Rodale Press, 1976.

Carper, Jean. *Stop Aging Now! The Ultimate Plan for Staying Young and Reversing the Aging Process.* New York: HarperCollins, 1995.

Castleman, Michael. *The Healing Herbs: The Ultimate*

Guide to the Curative Power of Nature's Medicines. New York: Bantam Books, 1991.

Castro, Miranda. *The Complete Homeopathy Handbook.* New York: St. Martin's Press, 1990.

Consumer Guide. The Women's Book of Home Remedies. Lincolnwood, Ill.: Publications International, 1994.

Dobelis, Inge N., ed. *Magic and Medicine of Plants.* Pleasantville, N.Y.: Reader's Digest, 1986.

Doress-Worters, Paula B., and Diana Laskin Siegal. *The New Ourselves, Growing Older: A Book for Women Over Forty.* New York: Touchstone Books, 1987.

Elkins, Rita. *The Complete Home Health Advisor: A Guide to Combining Standard Medical Treatments with Holistic Alternatives.* Pleasant Grove, Utah: Woodland Health Books, 1994.

Feltin, M. *A Woman's Guide to Good Health After 50.* Greenville, Ill.: Scott, Foresman, and Co., 1987.

Gach, Michael Reed. *Acupressure's Potent Points.* New York: Bantam Books, 1990.

Giller, Robert M., M.D, and Kathy Matthews. *Natural Prescriptions.* New York: Ballantine Books, 1994.

Griffith, H. W., M.D. *The Complete Guide to Medical Tests.* Tucson, Ariz.: Fisher Books, 1988.

Griffith, Winter H. *The Complete Guide to Vitamins, Minerals, Supplements, and Herbs.* Tucson: Fisher Books, 1988.

Haas, Elson M., M.D. *Staying Healthy with Nutrition.* Berkeley, Calif: Celestial Arts, 1992.

Hayflick, Leonard, Ph.D. *How and Why We Age.* New York: Ballantine Books, 1994.

Hendler, Sheldon Saul, M.D., Ph.D. *The Doctors' Vitamin and Mineral Encyclopedia.* New York: Fireside, 1990.

Houston, F. M., D.C., D.D., Ph.D. *The Healing Benefits of Acupressure.* New Canaan, Conn.: Keats Publishing, 1991.

Inglis, Brian, and Ruth West. *Alternative Health Guide.* New York: Knopf, 1992.

Kowalchik, Claire, and William H. Hylton, eds. *Rodale's Illustrated Encyclopedia of Herbs.* Emmaus, Pa: Rodale Press, 1987.

Law, Donald. *The Concise Herbal Encyclopedia.* New York: St. Martin's Press, 1973.

Lieberman, Shari, and Nancy Bruning. *The Real Vitamin and Mineral Book.* Garden City Park, N.Y.: Avery Publishing Group, 1990.

Lockie, Dr. Andrew. *The Family Guide to Homeopathy.* New York: Fireside, 1989.

Lockie, Dr. Andrew, and Dr. Nicola Geddes. *Homeopathy: The Principles and Practice of Treatment.* London: Dorling Kindersley, 1995.

Lust, John, N. D., and Michael Tierra, C. A., O.M.D. *The Natural Remedy Bible.* New York: Pocket Books, 1990.

Mabey, Richard, ed. *The New Age Herbalist.* New York: MacMillan Co., 1988.

Mayell, Mark, and the Editors of Natural Health Magazine. *The Natural Health First-Aid Guide.* New York: Pocket Books, 1994.

Mettler, Molly, M.S.W and Donald W. Kemper, M.P.H. *Healthwise for Life: Medical Self-Care for Healthy Aging.* Boise, Idaho: Healthwise, 1992.

Mindell, Earl, R.Ph., Ph.D. *Earl Mindell's Anti-Aging Bible.* New York: Fireside, 1996.

Murry, Michael, N.D., and Joseph Pizzorno, N.D. *Encyclopedia of Natural Medicine.* Rocklin, Calif.: Prima Publishing, 1991.

Natural Medicine Collective. *The Natural Way of Healing Stress, Anxiety, and Depression.* New York: Dell Publishing, 1995.

Ody, Penelope. *The Complete Medicinal Herbal.* London: Dorling Kindersley, 1993.

Olsen, Kristin Gottschalk. *The Encyclopedia of Alternative Health Care.* New York: Pocket Books, 1989.

Prevention Magazine Health Books. *The Doctors Book of Home Remedies.* New York: Bantam Books, 1990.

Prevention Magazine. *Hands-on Healing.* Emmaus, PA: Rodale Press, 1989.

Quillin, Patrick, Ph.D., R. D. *Healing Nutrients.* Chicago: Contemporary Books, 1987.

Silverman, Harold M., Parm.D., Joseph A. Romano,

Pharm.D., and Gary Elmer, Ph.D. *The Vitamin Book: A No-Nonsense Consumer Guide.* New York: Bantam Books, 1985.

Stanway, Dr. Andrew, with Richard Grossman. *The Natural Family Doctor.* New York: Fireside, 1987.

Stuart, Malcolm. *The Encyclopedia of Herbs and Herbalism.* New York: Crescent Books, 1979.

Weil, Andrew, M.D. *Health and Healing: Understanding Conventional and Alternative Medicine.* Boston: Houghton Mifflin, 1983.

Weil, Andrew, M.D. *Natural Health, Natural Medicine.* Boston: Houghton Mifflin, 1990.

Weiss, Gaea, and Shandor Weiss. *Growing and Using the Healing Herbs.* Emmaus, Pa.: Rodale Press, 1985.

Weiss, R. J., and G. Subak-Sharpe. *The Complete Guide to Health and Well-Being After 50.* New York: Columbia University School of Public Health, Random House, 1988.

Werbach, Melvyn, M.D. *Healing with Food.* New York: HarperPerennial, 1993.

Whitaker, Julian, M.D. *Dr. Whitaker's Guide to Natural Healing.* Rocklin, Calif.: Prima Publishing, 1995.

Young, Jacqueline. *Acupressure for Health.* San Francisco: Thorsons, 1994.

Appendix B: Organizations of Interest

For references to organizations on naturopathic medicine, see page 8; for those on herbal medicine, see pages 14–15; for those on diet and nutrition, see pages 34–35; for those on homeopathy, see page 58; and for organizations on acupressure, see pages 76–77. Other intradisciplinary organizations dealing with alternative medicine include:

Alliance for Alternatives in Health Care
P.O. Box 6279
Thousand Oaks, CA 91359-6279
(805) 494-7818

American Aging Association
2129 Providence Avenue
Chester, PA 19013-5506
(610) 874-7550

American Foundation for Alternative Health Care
25 Landfield Avenue
Monticello, NY 12701
(914) 794-8181

American Foundation of Traditional Chinese Medicine
505 Beach Street
San Francisco, CA 94133
(415) 776-0502

American Geriatrics Society
770 Lexington Avenue, Suite 300
New York, NY 10021
(212) 308-1414

American Holistic Medical Association
433 Front Street
Catasauqua, PA 18032
(610) 433-2448

Committee for Freedom of Choice in Medicine
1180 Walnut Avenue
Chula Vista, CA 91911
(619) 429-8200

Complementary Medicine Networking and Referral Service
4649 Malvern
Tucson, AZ 85711
(520) 323-6291

Well Spouse Foundation
610 Lexington Avenue, Suite 814
New York, NY 10022
(800) 838-0879

Index